——— REVISED EDITION ———

I Don't Remember Signing Up For CANCER!

SHERRY KARUZA WALDRIP

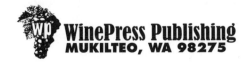
WinePress Publishing
MUKILTEO, WA 98275

The Wind Beneath My Wings
Words and Music by Larry Henley and Jeff Silbar
Warner House of Music

Illustrations by Judy Hanson Pregler

Printed in the United States of America

ISBN 1-57921-080-5
Library of Congress Catalog Card Number: 97-62404

To order additional copies of *I Don't Remember Signing Up For Cancer!* send $9.99 plus $3.95 to:
WinePress Publishing
P.O. Box 1406
Mukilteo, WA 98275
To order by credit card dial (800) 917-BOOK

I dedicate this book to my "Bosom Buddies" who have lost their battle with breast cancer but have won the war, because they are at home with their Lord and will suffer no more!

Gretchen Silverthorne

Betty Stafford

Bernice Schutz

Donna Mansell

Marjorie Cain

Liane Puseman

Deanna Reese

Margret Mazurek

Contents

Acknowledgments

Thank you, thank you, thank you to my family and friends for their loving support. Whenever I would get discouraged and say, "Get serious, I can't write a book!" these precious and faithful ones bullied me along. This book is theirs as well as mine. Thanks to:

JERRY . . . my wonderful husband, whose unyielding faith in me was a tremendous encouragement. I couldn't have faced cancer without his devotion and unwavering love, and I couldn't have written this book without his support and sacrifices. Thanks for still giving me palpitations after all these years, and for marrying me all over again on our 25th!

MICHAEL and DAVID . . . our incredible sons, whose loving concern for me during my cancer ordeal will forever touch my heart. They, too, constantly encouraged me as I wrote this book and were very patient with me during my preoccupation with this project, enduring it with minimal whining. Their pride in their mom touches my heart.

Our CARE GROUP . . . for their prayers and encouragement.

PATTY MINNIHAN . . . my precious pal, Perky Patty, a paragon of punctuation proficiency, painstakingly plucked me from paragraphical perils, page after page, while protecting my penned personality. Thank you, Patty, for the many hours you lovingly devoted to this book, and for your constant encouragement!

DR. ROBERT COOPER . . . for my beautifully reconstructed breast, for including me on some of his speaking engagements, and for taking the time out of his busy life to edit this book for medical accuracy.

RUSTY STANAWAY and KEN OLSEN . . . my favorite computer nerds, who always made themselves available to me, patiently helping me out of my computer scrapes (they didn't slap me even once!)

CLINT KELLY . . . My mentor and a wonderful author/speaker, who taught a class called "Writing to Make Them Laugh." He is a true "kindred spirit" who has taken me under his wing—encouraging me, praying with me, and guiding me all the way. Clint is the author of several adventure novels, including *The Landing Place* and *The Aryan*. And my favorite little book, *How to Win Grins and Influence Little People: Over 150 Fun and Creative Ways to Build Your Child's Self-esteem*.

JUDY HANSON PREGLER . . . for her cute and creative illustrations.

To my wonderful friends, who helped me face cancer with love, phone calls, cards, flowers, balloons, books, lunches, chocolate, evening meals, hugs and prayers.

A special thanks to: RONNIE BURGET, who pounded the doors of heaven faithfully praying for me, and who stepped in to take the maternal role when my mother couldn't be there. DONNA SWIFT and LYNN VINCENT, who rushed to my side as soon as I received the dreaded phone call, and who stuck like glue for the duration. Because of them I never had to go to a doctor's appointment alone. They invested many hours into loving me, crying with me, and making me laugh. While I wrote this book, they helped jog my memory and were diligent cheerleaders.

And most of all, to the LORD for His lovingkindness to me.

Foreword

If you are actually holding this book in your hands, you are witnessing a genuine miracle! The reason? I am a typical sanguine! Now, before you drop the book and cover your eyes in horror, believing this to be a scandalous confession, allow me to reassure you. In fact, a *sanguine* (a real official word, in the dictionary and everything) is one of the four personality temperaments. Two of the four are introverts, and the other two are extroverts. They each have both positive and negative traits. I'll offer a brief description:

- The "Perfect Melancholy": Analytical, talented, creative, idealistic, and perfectionistic, but can also be negative, moody, critical, and revengeful.
- The "Peaceful Phlegmatic": Calm, dependable, practical, patient, quiet, and witty, but on the down side, can be pessimistic, fearful, and unmotivated.
- The "Powerful Choleric": Decisive, optimistic, confident, organized, and motivational, but on the down side, can be very cruel, domineering, unemotional, proud, and inconsiderate.
- The "Popular Sanguine": Cheerful, curious, sincere, fun, friendly, compassionate, warm, and enthusiastic, but can also be undependable, restless, fearful, and undisciplined. (We can *sincerely* start a project with a bang, but often let it fizzle out and die.)

The undisciplined part is why it's a miracle you are holding this actual finished book in your hands. There were times when

I was dealing with writing a difficult or painful section of the book and someone would call with a more pleasant proposition. I was out'a there in a flash! But prayer and diligence finally won out, and *taaa daaa,* we have an actual book!

There are many books written on temperaments and personality types. One of my favorites, *Personality Plus,* was written by Florence Littauer, a fellow sanguine who is part choleric (which I'm sure helps with that disgusting "D" word: *discipline).* I can just imagine, however, the inner struggle between her sanguine and choleric sides:

"It's a great day to be productive and make important progress on the book," the choleric states firmly.

"I know, but there's excitement in the air, and I want to have fun today!" the sanguine counters, picking up the phone to call another fun-loving sanguine.

"No!" the choleric orders. "You will sit at the computer and write until your hands fall off!"

The sanguine spews, "Get a grip! Loosen up, you old party pooper. People who don't have fun get ugly and start smelling funny!"

"Very amusing," retorts the choleric. "Get busy, and remember, haste makes waste!"

What a battle it must have been. We all struggle with priorities, and eventually even sanguines will finish projects that are important to them.

This book was important to me. I had a burning desire to write it as an encouragement to women who have faced, are facing, or may face one of the most devastating diseases of our time, breast cancer. I felt driven to spread the news about the Free TRAM Flap, a wonderful, innovative, but little known reconstruction. I was also compelled to somehow express that humor can be an essential weapon when fighting illness—any illness. In addition, I wanted to pay tribute to my wonderful family and friends, who enfolded me in their loving arms and walked my difficult walk with me. Last, but certainly not least, writing this book is a small way that I might honor the God who is in the business of reconstructing hearts and lives.

I can certainly think of topics that would have been more fun to explore as I spread my wings to make my debut as an author. Nonetheless, it's the topic I got. But for the life of me, I don't remember signing up for cancer!

WARNING
READER DISCRETION ADVISED

I poke some fun at mammograms in the following chapter, but in no way is this meant to discourage anyone from getting a mammogram! This much-needed tool, used to detect cancer early, is essential, and although the test may be uncomfortable, cancer is even more so. Mammograms can detect cancer in the earliest of stages and can therefore save lives!

(Just don't do it when you're PMSing!)

Ode to a Mammogram

For years and years they told me, "Be careful of your breasts.
Don't ever squeeze or bruise them, and give them monthly tests."
So, I heeded all their warnings and protected them by law . . .
I guarded them carefully, and always wore a bra.
After thirty years of careful care, the doctor found a lump.
He ordered up a mammogram to look inside that clump.
"Stand up very close," she said, as she got my breast in line.
And, "Tell me when it hurts," she said. "Ah, yes! There, that's just fine."
When she stepped upon that pedal . . . I could not believe my eyes!
A plastic plate was pressing down. My boob was in a vise!!!
My skin was stretched 'n stretched from way up by my chin.
My poor breast was being smashed to Swedish pancake thin!
Oh! What a pang of pain I felt within its viselike grip!
A prisoner in this vicious thing, defenseless, there it sits!
"Take a deep breath," she said. Who does she think she's kidding?
My chest is smashed in her machine, and woozy I am getting.
"There! That was good," I heard her say as the room was slowly swaying.
"Now, let's get the other one." "Lord, have mercy," I was praying.
It squeezed me from up and down. It squeezed me from both sides.
Whatever is she doing to my tender little hide?
If I had no problem when I came in, I surely have one now.
If there had been a cyst in there, it would have gone ker-pow!
This machine was made by man, sweet revenge against his wife;
A female judge and jury would give him ten to life!

—Author unknown
Revised by Sherry Waldrip

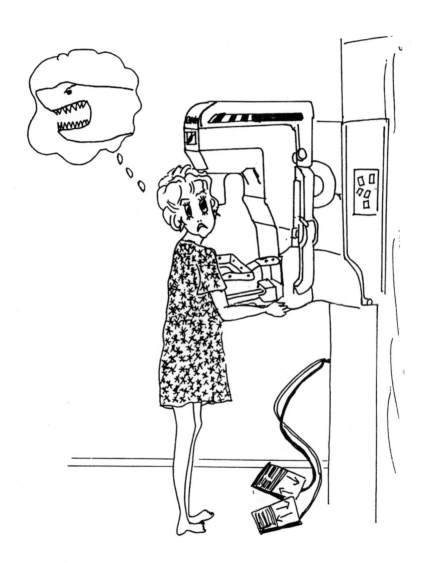

Chapter One
The Cruncher

It was as if I were being nagged by the media: Every time I picked up a magazine or newspaper, there was an article about breast cancer. When I turned on the television or radio, early detection through self-examination and mammography was being stressed. I had my first mammogram at age thirty-eight, and it wasn't too traumatic an ordeal. On my debut at Inland Imaging I joked with Jan the mammographer. As she led me to "The Cruncher," I could have sworn that I heard the theme song from the movie *Jaws* playing in the background. (She claimed she didn't hear it!) Paraphrasing Patsy Clairmont, one of my favorite writer-speaker-humorists, a mammography technician is someone who tries to make a saucer out of your cup! This is obviously a true statement. I was hoping my breasts would snap back into their natural state before I had to put on my bra and go home! If they didn't, just driving home could be a serious problem!

When she was done, she showed me the finished product. It didn't look much like a picture of a breast to me. I am a very sensitive person, however, and didn't want to hurt her feelings, so I asked for an 8x10 for my husband. She laughed, probably thinking that I had escaped from an asylum somewhere. We have since become friends, and now she is convinced that I did.

The mammogram turned out fine. I went on with my life, not really thinking too much about my breasts, except monthly, when PMS faithfully reminded me they were there and very much connected to my female plumbing. Every month I tell my husband, Jerry, "When I get to heaven, I'm decking Eve. This is all her fault. She and that wimpy husband! Furthermore, I hate snakes!"

I live in a household of men: Jerry, my extremely tolerant and loving husband; Michael, our firstborn, perfectionist son; and David, our very entertaining, lastborn son. They don't quite understand this woman stuff, but they are very patient with me. David has used it to his advantage, however. When grocery shopping he has grabbed a bag of M & M's or Hershey's Kisses, run them under my nose for the full effect of the aroma, and said, "You're MSPing Mom." (That's what he calls PMS.) "You really need these, don't you, Mom?!" I am ashamed to admit I have succumbed more often than not. Michael has bought me a big bag of M & M's and told me to save them for medicinal purposes. That has always seemed logical to me. They do, after all, resemble pills, so they *must* have some medicinal value.

DONNA'S ORDEAL

Donna, my dear and faithful friend, had lost her mother to breast cancer when she was fourteen. So when one of her mammograms revealed three calcifications, painful memories of childhood losses came flooding back. She was filled with fear over the possibility that her two daughters would feel the same pain that she and her sisters had experienced. At Donna's request, her family and friends were praying that when a needle localization was done prior to the biopsy, the calcifications would be gone.

I met Donna and her husband, Chuck, at Inland Imaging for the needle localization. In this procedure, a local anesthetic is used to numb the skin. The radiologist places a thin, hollow needle in the breast tissue, directing it toward the suspicious area seen on the x-rays. They then take two x-rays to ensure that the needle is as close to the suspicious area as possible. When they're sure that the needle is in the correct position, a skinny wire is threaded through the hollow needle. The radiologist then withdraws the needle, leaving the wire in place. Next, the patient is sent to surgery where the surgeon follows the wire to the area to be biopsied. The needle localization makes it possible for the surgeon to remove less breast tissue because the needle guides the surgeon to the suspicious area. It also makes it possible to biopsy those suspicious areas in the breast that cannot be felt.

While Donna was being x-rayed to determine where the needle would be placed, Chuck and I sat in the waiting room. Chuck asked me when my last mammogram was done. "I think it was about five years ago," I answered. He told me with a firm southern drawl, "Get yourself up to the front desk and make an appointment now!" It didn't occur to me to put up a fuss. I knew I was overdue. I obediently made my appointment for the following week and returned to my seat next to Chuck.

The technician came into the waiting room and asked for Chuck. I followed him as far as the doorway. The radiologist told Chuck that two of the calcifications had disappeared and the remaining one was too small to insert the needle. They called the surgeon and he canceled the biopsy. We were overwhelmed with joy! Donna and I shed tears of relief as we hugged each other and thanked the Lord for answering our prayers.

Judy, the mammographer who assisted the radiologist, was thrilled along with us. It was a happy morning, and we left floating on cloud nine, knowing that we had actually experienced a miracle.

The following week I rescheduled my mammogram, not wanting to experience "The Cruncher" during PMS soreness. I went in for my mammogram a week later. Judy and I talked about how rare it was for calcifications to just disappear as Donna's did. She told me how affected she was by Donna's and my devotion to each other and how the love and friendship we shared touched her heart. She laughed as I joked about "The Cruncher" throughout the exam and x-ray. When we were finished, she led me into a little room to watch a film about self-examination. "What! No popcorn?" I complained. Judy laughed, then disappeared. She reappeared after the film and told me I could get dressed and leave. The doctor's office would call me with the results. I sensed something. Judy was very professional, but I just knew in my gut that something was wrong.

I went home and busied myself, pushing my negative thoughts away. I reminded myself that there had never been a case of breast cancer in my family and that neither my doctor, Judy, nor I had felt a lump. It was just a routine procedure. Nothing to get worked up about. Statistics were in my favor.

Within a couple of hours I received a call from Dr. Sestero of Spokane Obstetrics and Gynecology. The x-ray showed a mass, a calcification, in one breast, so he recommended a biopsy. He suggested that I see Dr. Gary Matsumoto, the same surgeon who was to have done Donna's biopsy. Feeling numb, I hung up the phone. I can't say I was surprised because somehow I knew. I called Dr. Walter Balek, our family doctor, and Dr. Phil Monroe, a family friend. They both agreed that Dr. Matsumoto was a good choice.

It's amazing how a phone call can interrupt a silent afternoon in your home and permanently change your life. I was about to embark on an adventure, an episode in my life that every woman alive dreads.

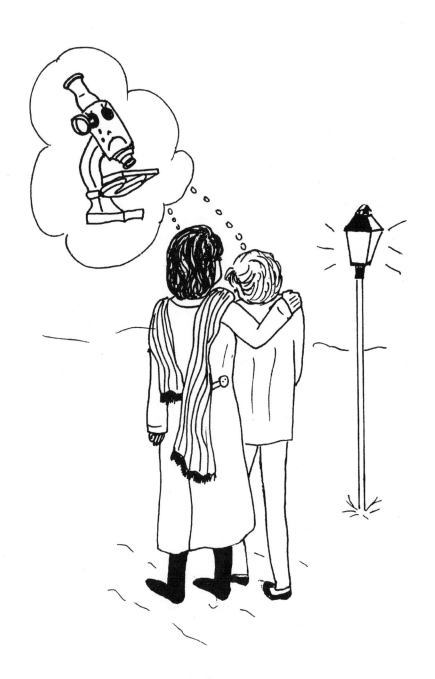

Chapter Two
The Biopsy Blues

November 12, 1990

Donna drove me to Dr. Matsumoto's office. As I waited in the examining room for him to arrive, I was hopeful that he would disagree with the radiologist and would say, "Oh, it's nothing, just a little dust that somehow got on the screen. Go home and eat chocolate."

He walked into the room looking so doctorly and serious that I couldn't bear it. His presence in the room was much too ominous for me to handle. I had to lighten the moment. I blurted out, "Your diplomas are all crooked. I hope you're better with a knife than you are with a hammer and nail." Caught off guard, he grinned and said, "I hope so too."

I managed to make the examination as lighthearted as possible. After examining me, he studied the x-rays and told me that the calcifications were clustered and a biopsy was necessary. My ears started ringing, and I was afraid I wouldn't remember or even compute what he was telling me. I asked if my friend Donna could come in while he explained everything.

Dr. Matsumoto was surprised to see Donna. They briefly spoke of her biopsy being canceled. As we all focused on my x-rays, he showed Donna and me the ugly intruder in my body. He explained the biopsy, then sent us out to schedule it.

I felt numb, and tears were rolling down my cheeks, so Donna took over. She stood by my chair, rubbing my back, and scheduled my biopsy. The earliest the biopsy could be done was the day before Thanksgiving. We closed the door behind us, and I dissolved into tears. Donna put her arm around me and we silently walked to the car.

November 20, 1990

The day before the biopsy, Donna took me in for the pre-surgery assessment, which includes blood work. Donna insisted on taking me. When she went through this herself, only weeks ago, it was her hardest day. I guess it's because the reality of it hits hard.

I have really wimpy veins. No one has ever been successful in drawing blood on the first stick. When a lab tech attempted to draw my blood while I was in labor with my first baby, more blood got on the sheets than in the tube! A very unpleasant experience. My husband was ready to wrap the IV pole around the frustrated blood tech's neck. This time was no different. The nurse couldn't get it her first time either. She sent me to the lab where that first attempt was successful. I was so grateful, Donna was afraid I would kiss the lab girl!

I talked to the anesthesiologist next. Rachel, my trusted counselor and my friend who had been helping me work through some childhood issues, had recommended that I have a general anesthetic instead of a local. I readily agreed. The thought of lying there awake, shooting the breeze with the surgical team while being fully aware of what they were doing and why, was too much for me. I preferred the "wake me when it's over" method. Rachel gave me the name of an anesthetic that minimized post-surgery nausea: Propafol. I presented a piece of paper with the name of the drug on it to the anesthesiologist, and he agreed. He was very kind and compassionate to me.

I became keenly aware of something very interesting to me on that day. At times the tension I experienced was so great that

I felt like a balloon that had been blown up so tightly it was in danger of exploding. I would crack a joke, feel a little less tension, and some of the pressure was relieved. I had always known that humor was helpful in relieving tension, but it became so real to me that day. Humor is my friend and has been all my life, especially during the tougher times. I appreciated this friend now more than ever.

I'm sure that people who don't know me well think, "The poor dear doesn't understand the seriousness of this situation." The truth is that I understand all too well. Therefore, I have to lighten the moment for myself, as well as for those around me.

I read somewhere that " . . . a keen sense of humor helps us to overlook the unbecoming, understand the unconventional, tolerate the unpleasant, overcome the unexpected, and outlast the unbearable." The prospect of breast cancer is at least four of those five, and I could not deal with it without the anesthetic of humor.

I once heard Chuck Swindoll, one of my favorite writer-speakers, say, "It's a bad thing to suppress laughter, because it goes back down and spreads your hips." Now I ask you, what sane person would choose gloom *and* wide hips?!

Norman Cousins in his book *Anatomy of an Illness* explains that humor is good not only for the spirit but for the body as well. It seems that it is a miracle drug with no side effects! This is not a new concept, however. Solomon said in Proverbs 17:22, "A cheerful heart is good medicine, but a crushed spirit dries up the bones" (NIV).

I much prefer laughter to tears, and even though at times it is difficult to pull it off, I am, for the most part successful.

At some point, however, we do need to get the tears out; it's the only honest thing to do. It's very cleansing and healing. I do not believe, as some do, that tears are a sign of weakness. They are a sign of strength. The Lord gave them to us for a reason. I believe that those who find pride in their ability to handle tragedy without grieving are motivated by the very thing that repulses them . . . fear. Fear of appearing weak.

23

One of the things I love most about our pastor, Tom Starr, is that he sheds tears over his congregation, and Tom is one of the strongest men I know.

I believe that our Lord also feels our pain. Psalms 56:8 says, "You have seen me tossing and turning through the night. You have collected all my tears and preserved them in your bottle! You have recorded every one in your book" (LB). He cares!

One day, however, we won't have to deal with pain. Revelation 21:4 says, "He will wipe away all tears from their eyes and there shall be no more death, nor sorrow, nor crying, nor pain. All of that has gone forever" (LB). This is a promise to believers—something to look forward to!

November 21, 1990

Donna met Jerry and me at Inland Imaging and waited with Jerry, just as I had waited with her husband, Chuck, only weeks earlier. I went in for the needle localization (described in chapter one). Donna told me that she had been praying the same for me as she had for herself, that when they took the x-ray to determine where to place the needle, the calcifications would be gone. She was sure that my biopsy would be canceled just as hers had been. We had gone to the women's Bible study at the church the morning before. There the women prayed that the Lord would take the calcifications away. As the procedure continued, it became apparent that the Lord had different plans for me than what we had hoped.

The tension of the moment was getting to me, big time. The doctor had me in "The Cruncher." My back was hurting, both from the contorted position I was in and from being so uptight. My balloon was tensing up.

"So, are you a boob man, or what?" I couldn't believe I said that to a total stranger!

He just smiled and replied, "No, actually I'm a leg man."

What a relief! I thought. *He wasn't offended. I think I'll just be quiet now. Yes, that's what I'll do. At least for the next procedure I'll be unconscious. I behave much better when I'm unconscious.*

24

I hadn't planned on looking, but I did. It was strange seeing six inches of wire sticking out of my breast with a little tiny drop of blood emerging from beneath. They put a gown over me and told me not to move my arm for fear of moving the wire. They escorted me out to Jerry and Donna, who drove me across the parking lot to the hospital. Jerry parked the car.

"Do we really have to do this?" I cried, already knowing the answer to my question. Jerry and Donna lovingly tried to comfort me as they gently helped me out of the car, taking care not to dislodge the wire.

I wasn't given anything to relax me prior to being wheeled into surgery. I sure could have used something. I lay there waiting for my turn on the table. The anesthesiologist to whom I had spoken the day before was there, and I was happy to see a familiar face. I told him that since I was already there and all, they might just as well go ahead and do a face lift and tummy tuck and get it all done in one shot. He said this wasn't the right day for the "blue light special." I heard a woman's voice on the other side of a screen say, "You mean this isn't K-Mart?" I think she was also awaiting the knife.

Not that I was in any hurry, but it was finally my turn. The table was so hard, and the light above was so bright. Everyone wore masks, and I was terrified. I said, "You know, I hardly ever lay on a table naked in front of men."

One of the masked men patted my arm and said, "Well, this will be a new experience for you."

I could tell by his eyes he was smiling. I thought, *Hardly ever! Why did I say that? I made it sound like it was something I do occasionally but not very often. The truth is I've never had an experience like this in my life!* They slipped me a Mickey, and I was out . . .

I vaguely remember recovery. As the nurses gently cared for me, they joked with each other. It was the day before Thanksgiving and they were playfully looking forward to the holiday. I was too out of it to play along. I hate it when fun is happening and I'm not in the middle of it! It was so difficult to wake up.

Following recovery, as we came off the elevator, I saw Jerry, Donna, Lynn, Mary, Pam, and Laura. I didn't know they would all be there. Lynn, my zany partner in lunch and lunacy, claims that as they wheeled me off the elevator I was doing the beauty queen wave with a spacy look on my face and saying, "They loved me!" Lynn is a sanguine and I think she made it up!

They sat me in a chair similar to a dentist's chair, which I didn't much care for because I wanted to lie down. The reason for the chair is to help you wake up faster so they can kick you *out*. That's why they call it *Out*-patient surgery. It sure made me want to get *out* so I could go home and lie down. I was pretty spacy—any kind of drug or medication seems to hit me hard.

While I was in recovery, Dr. Matsumoto had called down to say that the suspicious area just looked like fatty tissue. Everyone was relieved—to say the least. Jerry took me home, fixed me some soup, and I rested until bedtime. The phone rang a lot. I heard Jerry telling the callers that it looked good and I would be "back at it" in no time.

Thanksgiving 1990

Feeling optimistic about the biopsy, we spent Thanksgiving with friends. I pretty much just sat, visited, and got pampered. When Jerry changed the dressing that night, I felt sad that my breast was bruised and dented; but I was thankful I had it, and it looked like I would be able to keep it. I fell asleep in Jerry's arms, truly thankful on that Thanksgiving.

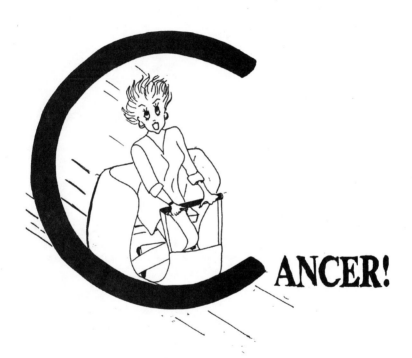

C ANCER!

Chapter Three

The "C" Word and My Roller Coaster Ride

The Monday after Thanksgiving, I was busy baking cookies when the phone rang. It was Dr. Matsumoto calling with the results of my biopsy. He used the word *cancer* and my name in the same sentence. I was stunned. It seemed like he was talking too fast, or maybe I was listening too slowly. Nonetheless, I knew that what he was saying wasn't computing. He used words like *Ductal Carcinoma In-situ*. In-situ! Wouldn't you know, *I'd* get a disease that sounds like a martial art?

"But you said it looked good . . . that it looked like fatty tissue," I pleaded.

He said, "I know. I was surprised too. I had them run the test twice, to be sure before I called you."

"What do we do now?" I asked.

He replied, "Well, it's in the very early stages, and with a mastectomy, the cure rate is high— 99 percent."

The word *mastectomy* sent a shiver up my spine. I scribbled down what he said on paper, thinking it all would make some sense later.

I hung up the phone in shock. I tried to call Donna, but crying and shaking, I kept pushing the wrong numbers on the phone. Finally, I got through. I somehow got the words out of my mouth, and she was just as shocked as I. Next, I called my mother in California. She was concerned because I was alone. I told her Donna was on her way. By the time I got off the phone, Donna was by my side. She hugged me and cried with me. She finished baking the cookies I had started, cleaned up the mess, and fixed some soup. Stunned by the bad news, I had overlooked lunch. It felt strange to have another woman in my kitchen waiting on me; but, something told me she needed to do it, and at that moment, I needed to be taken care of. Jerry called. He never calls during the day. Working in new construction, he is rarely near a phone. He rushed home to my side. His arms felt so safe. Can this really be happening to me, to us?

Lynn got back to me as soon as she heard the message I had left on her machine. "The doctor just called with the results." I cried.

"Oh crap!" she exclaimed. "I'll be right there!" Within minutes she rushed through our front door saying, "Don't worry about a thing, I'm a firstborn. I can fix this!" Lynn, as always, lightened a very heavy moment.

Anyone who has read Kevin Lehman's *Birth Order Book* knows that firstborns like Lynn and myself are convinced it is our job to fix things: tidy up the messy things in life and make them right. We firstborns constantly run up against the brick walls of life; but, we are a hardy breed, and tenacity is our middle name. Lynn and I have laughed and teased each other about this for years, so it seemed appropriate that she should bring up the superhuman skills of a firstborn at a time like this.

Just one year ago at this same time of year, Lynn lost her mother to this horrible monster called cancer. Now, here was another personal attack from an enemy she hated! She brought with her all of the information she had collected during her mother's illness, including the 1-800-4CANCER information hotline. Donna called and requested that they send me all the current information about breast cancer and treatment.

Jerry called Dr. Matsumoto and listened as he explained my type of cancer. *Ductal carcinoma* meant that my cancer was in the milk duct, and *in-situ* meant it was in the very beginning stages.

I had time to decide what I wanted to do, to "get all my ducks in a row," as Dr. Matsumoto said, but I shouldn't take too long. After all, we were dealing with cancer here.

Dr. Matsumoto said I was "*lucky*" that we caught my cancer so early. "Why don't I *feel* lucky? Why am I so sick to my stomach?"

Jerry left to pick up David at basketball practice and told him on the way home. To conceive that his mom had cancer was so difficult for my tenderhearted fifteen-year-old macho man, my last born, my clown. He just sat very still on the couch, his arm tenderly around me, staring silently at the carpet.

Jerry went next door to tell Gary and Peggy the results of my biopsy. Their daughters, Terri and Amy, are the same ages as our two sons. Amy and David were in diapers when their family moved next door to us. Now the kids were teenagers. We have raised our kids together and are very close. In sharing this experience called "life," we have always been able to count on each other for anything. They came home with Jerry. Peggy was crying; she said she was angry! I wondered if anger was what I was feeling. "Am I angry?" I asked myself. "I'm not sure yet. I probably should be. I know I feel numb. Numb and afraid."

Pastor Rich, our music minister, his wife, Marge, and Dr. Phil came over. Just a few days earlier we had spent Thanksgiving together and had all felt so positive about the outcome of the biopsy. This time we were together for them to love and encourage us. We laughed, ate cookies, shared our hearts, and finally prayed together. It was a special time with friends.

Bedtime came, Jerry and I cried in each others arms, and I fell asleep praying, "Oh Lord, I'm so scared!"

The next day several of my friends came over to spend the day with me. I think back on it now and realize how loving and thoughtful it was for them to want to be with me, to show their love and support. It could have been almost like a party had it not been for the dreaded word *cancer* over our heads, the gruesome word *mastectomy* on our minds. They all knew it could happen to them as well as to me. It seems like breast cancer spins a roulette wheel to choose it's victims. It's a gamble, the flip of a cruel coin. Breast cancer is a random killer. It knows no ethnic, religious, or socioeconomic boundaries. It seems nothing I did caused it, and there was nothing I could have done to prevent it. One out of every nine women gets it . . .seems kind of grim.

Jerry and I went to a radiologist to see if radiation would be an option, a way to avoid the mastectomy. As we sat quietly in the waiting room, I was having an ugly pity party in my mind. Jerry, who seems to always expect the best from me, would have been shocked. I was so angry that I was there. Everyone else in the waiting room was elderly, and most of them had oxygen tanks with them. I made cold judgements that they had probably caused their own cancer by smoking all their lives. I was young. I hadn't done anything to cause this. Why was I here among these people? It seemed likely that they had destroyed their own bodies; they knew the risks and made the choice to smoke. What had I done? Nothing!

Then, at the height of my pity party, a little girl about nine years old walked in with her mother. She had obviously lost her hair through chemotherapy. As she curled up next to her mother, I felt ashamed of what was in my heart.

Suddenly my pity party ended. *Okay, Lord,* I thought, *I get it. Cancer doesn't care about age!* Which, of course, I already knew. The Lord sent that little angel to show me that I was not the only blameless victim of this hateful disease, and I was certainly not the youngest. Second, how did I dare judge the cause of the other patients' illness. I was thankful that they couldn't read my mind. I asked the Lord to forgive me for my ugly attitude and prayed for the other patients, especially for that sweet little girl who, without knowing it, ministered to me. I guess the numbness was wearing off, and this was my first glimpse of the anger that my neighbor, Peggy, had felt that first night.

The doctor read the report, examined me, then explained to us that he agreed with Dr. Matsumoto. A mastectomy was the best option with the highest cure rate. This was *not* music to my ears, since I was hoping and praying that we could find a way to get rid of the cancer, yet somehow avoid the mastectomy—that radiation would be my answer. Before leaving, we spent some time talking to a nurse named Marcy. She was very kind and asked if she could have a nurse she knew call me. Sylvia had been in my shoes just a year earlier. I eagerly agreed.

Michael was away at college in California. We tried to avoid telling him about my cancer, at least while he was in the middle of finals. In a couple of weeks he would be home, and then we could sit down as a family and work it through together. I should have known better. He sensed something was wrong over the phone. We had previously told him about the biopsy, believing the results were favorable. He kept asking questions, and we tried to answer them without using the word *cancer*. He was becoming frustrated by our vagueness and just blurted out, "Is it cancer Mom?" I didn't answer right away. "Mom, answer me!"

"Yes, Honey, it is, but it's in the early stages and curable. . . I'll be fine. Try not to worry. You need to get through your finals." I tried to comfort and reassure him.

"I wish I was home with you, Mom." (He's a firstborn and wants to fix it.)

"You will be home for Christmas soon. Like I said, the cancer is in the very early stages, and it's the slow-growing kind. I don't have to rush into surgery. I can wait until after Christmas. We will be together soon, so try to concentrate on your schoolwork. You have to pass those finals."

"I can't wait to hug you, Mom!" he said with love and concern.

When we hung up, I prayed that the Lord would comfort him. I wasn't too concerned. Michael had made so many wonderful friends at the college. The chorale music group he was in was so much like a family to him, and I was certain he would have lots of love and support.

JOURNAL ENTRIES

Tuesday, December 4, 1990
"Dear Lord,

Today was a terrible, no good, very bad day! I didn't sleep well last night. Kept dreaming about cancer (wonder why). The nurse that Marcy told us about called. I couldn't believe the parallels in our lives. We were the same age, her husband sounded a lot like Jerry, she had two girls the same age as my two boys, we had the same kind of cancer in the same breast, and best of all, we both love You, Lord. She was able to minister to me on every level. Lord, sometimes You are such a kick in the pants. You planned that one pretty slick!

She explained everything I would go through medically, from the mastectomy to the reconstruction. What she had to say about the reconstruction was discouraging to me. I thought the implant would be put in when they did the mastectomy. Sylvia explained that they put only the tissue expander behind the muscle at the same time as the mastectomy. Then they build it up gradually to the desired size, which takes several months and several trips to the plastic surgeon's office. It seems it will be months before I feel and look whole again. I'm having such a difficult time readjusting my thinking.

We went to David's basketball game tonight. I get such kick out of watching him play. Afterward, we stayed for half of the varsity game. I have been told the odds are strongly in my favor, but cancer is so scary! Will I be around when David plays varsity? Please let me, Lord! I'm not afraid to die; according to the Bible, heaven is a much better place. It's just that I have such love for my family of men. I can't leave them—not yet, Lord!

Rachel called tonight. She is glad I'm shedding some tears, letting my frustrations out. This sad Sherry seems so unnatural to me. Have I lost my *sanguineness?* Where did my joy go? I would rather be Sherry the Clown. I know her better and like her so much more. She's my friend. I'm not comfortable with this new companion named Despair! Will I ever feel happy and carefree again? Will I ever again laugh and make others laugh? Is Sherry the Sanguine gone forever? I know you see the whole picture, Lord, and I see only a small part, frame by frame. Please help me to trust you. Please help me feel your presence, your comfort, your peace. Please, at the very least, help me get a good night's sleep!"

Wednesday, December 5, 1990
"Dear Lord,

Today was a good day. I slept very well last night. Thank you! I received many encouraging phone calls today. I spent the afternoon with Lynn. She is such good medicine for me. We laughed a lot, and I think we covered every subject in the world (with our own peculiar bent, of course!). A little of the sanguine popped out today with Lynn; maybe I *will* have joy again. It's possible there's hope for me after all!

Sylvia called. I can't wait to meet her. I believe she is a gift from You, Lord. Thank you!

Jerry has been so good at making me feel cherished. I think this nightmare has made us closer than ever. I love him so much. Lying beside him at night is such a gift. I'm so thankful he chose me to spend his life with!"

Thursday, December 6, 1990
"Dear Lord,

Jerry came home this morning with a migraine. This is taking its toll on him too. He has been so strong for me, but some-

35

times I think this is even harder on him. To watch me struggle through this experience while feeling so helpless must be horrid for him. He has always tried his best to protect and shield me from harm. This time he can't to a thing. He must be very angry. For some reason he craves potato soup after a migraine, so I peeled potatoes and made soup before leaving for Christian Women's Club prayer coffee.

It was good to be with the board members again. Torchy, our prayer advisor, had a special prayer time for me. Bless her, Lord. She is such a faithful friend and a real prayer warrior. They all think I am doing so well—if they only knew the despair and sadness I feel at times. The pity parties, the fear of my husband being repulsed by me (although if he were, I know he would hide it). Will I feel sexy after the amputation of my breast? Will I still playfully tease him? Will I continue to write provocative notes to slip into his pockets or his lunch? Or will I shut down sexually and start dressing in the closet? After all these years, I would rather not be inhibited and withdraw from my husband, Lord! But how will I help it? I won't be the same!

I came home from the meeting and had some soup with Jerry. We took a nap together, and he felt good enough to go back to work. I finally felt up to some housework and started downstairs. It will take days to get this place back in shape! I have really neglected my home in this new adventure.

David came home from basketball practice with two dislocated knees. He's really hobbling around. What a family! David's knee, Jerry's migraine, and my boob! Hope Michael is doing better at college than we are at home! Thank you, Lord, for two good nights' sleep!"

Friday, December 7, 1990
"Dear Lord,

Today was a pretty good day. Ronnie came over and did some housework for me while I did her Christmas letter on the computer. She sings while she cleans. I do that sometimes, but I only sound that good in my dreams! Between the two of us we got the house back in shape. It was so good to finally give some attention to my home again!

Jerry had a root canal this morning—such fun! We always have something interesting going on around here. I was mostly up today, just a few moments of sadness. Dad called to check on me. He's getting stronger from his surgery."

Saturday, December 8, 1990
"Dear Lord,

Today was a real roller coaster ride: up one minute, down the next. We had a rehearsal for the Christmas cantata this morning. I came home feeling really down. Realizing that Christmas is coming regardless of my state of mind, I decorated the house. I listened to Christmas music, desperately trying to get into the holiday spirit.

We had dinner with Ron and Connie to celebrate Connie's birthday. I finally got to meet Sylvia. She and her husband, Clee, are the organizers of The Master's Table. They meet in the banquet room of a downtown restaurant every Saturday night. It's a place where you can enjoy a candlelight dinner and listen to Christian musicians. We had a lovely dinner and enjoyed a wonderful country western group.

The highlight for me though was meeting Sylvia. We have had many telephone conversations, so it was wonderful to finally meet her face to face. When the evening was over, Sylvia handed me a package, not to be opened until I got home. What she didn't know, however, was that when it comes to presents, I am still five years old. Everyone knows that a five-year-old can't possibly sit with a beautifully wrapped package on her lap for an entire twenty-minute ride home. Of course not! While Jerry and Ron scraped the snow off the car windows, Connie and I ripped that sucker open in record time! It was a wonderful centerpiece called "Celebrations of the Seasons" that had four candles and wooden figures to be changed seasonally: hearts for Valentines Day, shamrocks for St. Patrick's Day, bunnies for Easter, tulips for springtime and summer; jack-o-lanterns for Halloween, fall leaves for autumn, turkeys for Thanksgiving, and angels and Christmas trees for Christmas. On the card Sylvia had written:

> *Dear Sherry,*
>
> *Keep in mind that when the Lord chooses to use human vessels to perform His work, we must patiently and prayerfully allow that process to unfold under His guiding hand.*
>
> *By the time you bring out the tulips, you and He will have emerged on the back side of all this!*
>
> *Wishing you and your family the Lord's peace this Christmas,*
>
> Sylvia

I wanted to run back inside and thank her with a big hug. But then she would have known I was a naughty five-year-old who couldn't wait twenty minutes to open her wonderful gift."

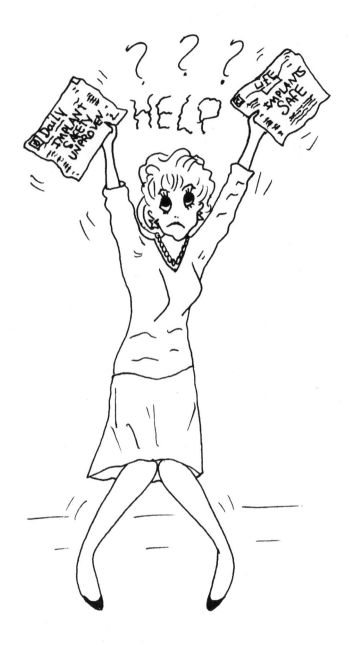

Chapter Four

The Implant Impact

Jerry's dad called in the morning. I have loved him like a father since the first time Jerry took me to his parents' Oregon ranch in 1968. He is a strong and tall man with beautiful white hair, a great sense of humor, and a twinkle in his eye. We love to tease each other, and he tells me I make the best apple pie in the entire country. This phone call seemed different. He was concerned. He had seen *Face to Face* with Connie Chung the night before, a program about implants. I told him I hadn't watched it yet but had taped it and planned to watch it that night. He insisted I not have an implant. "Just do without," he said.

"I don't know if I could handle that, Dad."

"Sure you could," he said. "Just get one of those things to wear in your bra. No one will know but you and Jerry. It would be better than something that will make you sick!"

We hung up and I felt a cloud over my head. Dad had never talked to me like that before. I can see why his three kids turned out so well—he has a way of making you want to do the right thing. I felt like what he wanted me to do was the right thing. I also felt like the right thing wouldn't work for me. Was it vanity? No, I think vanity is not wanting to leave the house on a bad hair day. I think it has more to do with wanting to feel whole, not wanting to be robbed of what society has taught me is part of my womanhood, part of what makes me desirable to my husband.

I was a late bloomer, slow to mature. My friends were rude enough to show signs of womanhood before me! I remember, as a preteen, stuffing my bathing suit with Kleenex and coming out to Crow Canyon Pool thinking I looked like Marilyn Monroe and just knowing that everyone was stunned by my shapely beauty, that Hollywood would be calling soon. My dad caught up with me and told me to march back in the bathroom and take whatever I stuffed in there *out!* My thoughts of being a bathing beauty were gone, dashed forever on that day many years ago. I had been so angry with him and told him so a few years ago. He said, "Honey, they were lumpy, and one was higher than the other; I couldn't let you strut around looking like that!" It's probably a good thing he caught up with me before I got into the pool!

Now, I had another father telling me that I didn't need this evidence of womanhood. Is that what my Heavenly Father was telling me too? Don't fathers care about their daughters feeling like women? Didn't it matter to them that I wanted to feel sexy, whole, complete?

Society's fascination with women's breasts is not exactly something new. In the Song of Solomon, written almost three thousand years ago, Solomon repeatedly mentions the beauty of his beloved's breasts. I'm pretty sure Jerry has never referred to my breasts as the "twin fawns of a gazelle," but he has definitely referred to them with appreciation—and I felt insecure at the thought of losing one. I had to face the amputation of one of my "fawns," and the thought of no reconstruction was devastating to me!

I couldn't bear to watch Connie Chung's program alone, so I waited for Jerry to come home. I did the dinner dishes, then we settled on the couch in the family room to watch it. I cuddled next to Jerry, clinging tightly to a pillow while I listened in horror. As these women unfolded their nightmares, I began to have one of my own. I felt physically ill as I heard them describe their symptoms: swollen glands, flu-like symptoms, joint pain, fatigue, sore throats, mouth ulcers, hair loss, rashes, even Lupus. They called it Silicone Associated Disease. In some cases, silicone was found in almost every part of the body. Women who had had implants for augmentation (breast enlargement) said that when they had their implants removed they ended up looking almost like they'd had a bilateral mastectomy. The women who had implants for reconstruction following a mastectomy felt as if they had gone through the horror of the mastectomy twice.

I was sure that the physical and emotional pain these women expressed was heartbreaking to any woman who watched. But to someone who was facing this very thing in a couple of weeks, it was devastating. The anxiety I felt was overwhelming. I wanted to throw something across the room. My love for Jerry, knowing his pain and feelings of powerlessness over this enemy attacking his wife both physically and emotionally, overruled my frustration. I couldn't, wouldn't, make it worse for him by acting out the rage I felt escalating inside of me. I just sat there and silently wept as he tenderly held me. It appeared that my only hope of looking and feeling whole again after the amputation of my breast was gone. Jerry was heartbroken by my despair, and as he held me, he again reassured me that it didn't matter—he loved *me*, not my breasts. He married Sherry, the whole person; he didn't marry a breast. He would *always* love me, no matter what!

Bless his heart. He said all the right things. We went up to bed and he held me while he prayed for me. As I tried to fall asleep in his arms, my feelings of grief and hopelessness were overwhelming. I had crazy thoughts of refusing the mastectomy. "Cancer is a death sentence anyway; if I'm going to die, I might as well die in one piece instead of carved up like the Thanksgiving turkey we had just days ago!" There was so much going on in the roller coaster of my mind. If I could only turn it off for a while and sleep. I felt so weary. Sleep would turn off the pain, at least for a while, at least until morning.

"What am I going to do Lord?" I prayed in my heart. "Please help me. I know I have to have the mastectomy, and of course I will. But I want to feel whole!"

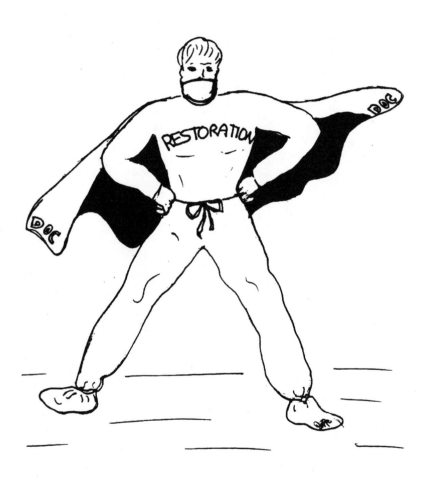

Chapter Five
Reconstruction Is Alive and Well

The next morning I was exhausted. Not sleeping well really takes its toll. I fixed breakfast and packed lunches, just as I do every morning. After Jerry left for work and David for school, I showered and cleaned up the breakfast dishes. I was baking Christmas cookies when the doorbell rang. I wasn't expecting anyone, but welcomed the diversion. It was Pam; she attends the same church we do. I expressed the anguish I felt after watching *Face to Face*.

She listened sympathetically, then told me that although she didn't remember where she learned about it she thought there was a procedure where a plastic surgeon could use your tummy to build a new breast. Her visit felt like a visit from an angel. She wasn't even out of the driveway before I was on the phone to the cancer hotline, 1-800-4CANCER, the number Lynn had left for me.

The woman I talked to was very helpful. That particular reconstruction, she explained, is called the "TRAM Flap." She told me everything she knew about the procedure, then added that Dr. Patrick Maxwell, a plastic surgeon in Nashville, had published an article about it. I hung up and immediately dialed information in Nashville to get Dr. Maxwell's phone number.

I called and talked to his office nurse. "Women love it!" she exclaimed. "They awaken from surgery with a nicely shaped, natural looking breast." She suggested that I come to Nashville. "It's a more specialized surgery and not many plastic surgeons do it." I thanked her, but told her I needed to try to find someone closer to home. She cautioned me to call only "board certified" plastic surgeons and to inquire whether they had experience with the TRAM Flap procedure. I thanked her for the encouraging information. She wished me luck as we hung up.

As I put the phone back on the receiver, I realized that I was excited and hopeful for the first time in weeks. I immediately prayed and thanked the Lord for the gift of hope, then asked Him to please help me find a plastic surgeon close to home. I was willing to go to Portland or Seattle if needed, but, I prayed, "Lord, please, please, please help me find a plastic surgeon who does this surgery, and let him be in Spokane—and thank you, Lord, for this new hope I feel!"

On my second call I hit the jackpot! I had reached Dr. Robert Cooper who had been in town only a few months. I made an appointment to meet with him on the following Monday. When I hung up the phone, my heart was filled with such gratitude to the Lord for answering my prayers! Within a couple of hours I had gone from hopeless and defeated to hopeful and ecstatic. I called Lynn and Donna who were both thrilled, not only for me but because there was an alternative to implants!

I called Gloris, a friend of Sylvia's who had been ministering to me in many ways. Gloris attends Sylvia's church, is a nurse in the office of a general surgeon, and is a breast cancer survivor herself. Gloris had a calming effect on me as she and I spent much time on the phone. Sylvia and Gloris continued to encourage and minister to me in a way that only women who have faced breast cancer can. I like to call the women who have faced this mutual challenge my "Bosom Buddies." We are bosom buddies not only for the obvious reason but also for the way we take each other into our hearts. It's a real sisterhood—certainly not a chosen one, but a sisterhood nonetheless!

Gloris was intrigued as I explained the TRAM Flap, intrigued both as a surgeon's nurse and as a woman who had been where I was about to tread. I asked her to go with Jerry and me for my first appointment with Dr. Cooper. Both her professional and personal opinions were very important to me.

It was amazing to realize that just the night before I had fallen asleep crying out to God from the bottom of the pit of despair. Tonight I was on the mountaintop of hope, rejoicing that my prayers had been answered. The God who spoke the world into being heard the groanings and pleas of a grieving woman in Spokane, Washington. And even though my prayers were completely self-focused and of no significance or spiritual value to the world, He looked down in His mercy and saw Sherry Lynn lying in her husband's arms, with a broken heart. I was reminded of the words of a song: "His eye is on the sparrow, and I know He watches me." How hopeless it seems to me to believe life is an evolution—from goo to you, by way of the zoo! How comforting it is to *know* that we have a creator, a Heavenly Father who watches over us and that *His* heart is broken over *our* heart that's broken! My God and Heavenly Father knew my longing to be, and feel, whole as a woman. He knew that I was heartsick about the loss of my breast and that it seemed hopeless to long for wholeness through reconstruction. Proverbs 13:12 says: "Hope deferred makes the heart sick, but a longing fulfilled is a tree of life" (NIV). I felt revived and strengthened. I felt life again!

When Jerry came home from work, I attacked him at the door with my exciting news. He was thrilled to see me happy and excited about something again. During our marriage, it was customary for me to greet him at the door with a kiss and hug and excitement that he was home. Through this experience of cancer, however, I had lost my joy, and unfortunately, he usually had to come through the house to find me, then try in vain to cheer me up. He was delighted to be attacked at the door with the smiles and kisses of an enthusiastic wife once again. (My poor husband. Here I was dragging him along on my roller coaster ride of emotions, and he doesn't even *like* roller coasters!)

It was handy that this exciting news came on a Wednesday. I remembered vaguely that on the night of my diagnosis, Dr. Phil mentioned a new plastic surgeon in town who was building quite a reputation for himself: very skilled, very personable. Phil hadn't met him yet, but as a physician, he was impressed with what he had heard through the medical grapevine. I had been in a fog that night and couldn't remember the plastic surgeon's name. I couldn't wait to get to choir practice to find out if Dr. Cooper was the one of whom Phil had spoken.

Before I saw Phil, I saw my friend Joannie, an orthopedic nurse. Of course, I told her my good news! She smiled and told me Dr. Cooper had done a skin graft on a patient who had been in a motorcycle accident. It was the best skin graft she had ever seen, pink and healthy looking. Joannie was impressed with his work, and I was elated!

I grabbed Phil as soon as I could and asked the question on my heart. He said, "Yes, it was Dr. Cooper I was talking about." I reacted as any mild-mannered sanguine would, I jumped up and down, threw my arms around him and squealed, "That's wonderful!" He looked a little puzzled, although I don't know why. He was certainly used to me by then!

I felt, however, that I should probably explain my outburst. He listened intently as I explained what I knew about the procedure at that point, which wasn't a lot. He looked concerned and said, "Does it have a blood supply? If it doesn't, the tissue will die."

What a party pooper, I thought! "Then it must!" I responded. "I see him Monday and I'll let you know."

I felt like Scarlet O'Hara in *Gone With the Wind* when she said, "I won't think about that today. I'll think about that tomorrow!" I wasn't going to let anything spoil my good mood. It seemed like forever since I'd had a good mood, and it felt *good*!

On Thursday, *December 13,* we had our Christmas Brunch for Christian Women's Club and it was great!

Dr. Matsumoto had set up a reconstruction consultation for me weeks before with Dr. Gerald Olmsted, a plastic surgeon. Although I had planned to see Dr. Cooper on Monday, I decided to keep my appointment with Dr. Olmsted. I was curious as to what he thought about the TRAM Flap, not that he could discourage me. It was snowing and the roads were slick, so Torchy and her husband, Chuck, drove me downtown.

Gloris, my new friend, informant, and encourager, worked in the same medical building where Dr. Olmsted had his office. I made arrangements to meet with her for the first time, after hours of telephone conversations. Torchy and I followed Gloris to an examining room so we could have some privacy as we talked. She showed us her implant, saying she was happy with it and had no problems. It looked great! I told her the shape of the implant was different from the shape of my breast. I was concerned about having a mismatched set. She assured me that the plastic surgeon can do reconstruction on the healthy breast to match them up again. I reminded her of my appointment with Dr. Cooper, and she assured me she would be there. She was interested for personal and professional reasons and wanted to share the information with the surgeon she worked for.

Torchy and I then headed for Dr. Olmsted's office. There the nurse led us to a room to view a slide presentation: pictures of women after their mastectomies, both before and after reconstruction. My heart was broken for the faceless women on the slides—amputation seems like such a brutal way to treat a disease. I had a difficult time dealing with myself being in their position, as I'm sure *they* did! I became even more convinced that this TRAM Flap procedure was what I wanted.

After the film, we were taken to an examining room, and soon Dr. Olmsted came in. We exchanged courteous greetings. He looked me in the eye and said, "Sherry, what do you want to do?" I looked right back at him with a determination that surprised me and said, "I want the TRAM Flap!"

He seemed surprised. Knowing he didn't do the TRAM Flap, I fully expected him to try to discourage me, and I was ready for the challenge.

He examined me and said, "From what I know of the TRAM Flap, you look like a good candidate. Although I have watched the surgery, I have never been involved. If Dr. Cooper agrees that you are a good candidate, and if he doesn't already have someone to assist him, would you tell him I would love to assist him in your surgery?"

I happily agreed and was thrilled by his reaction! I also took his positive attitude as an affirmation that this was the right road for me to pursue. Now I was even more anxious to meet this new man in town, Dr. Robert Cooper.

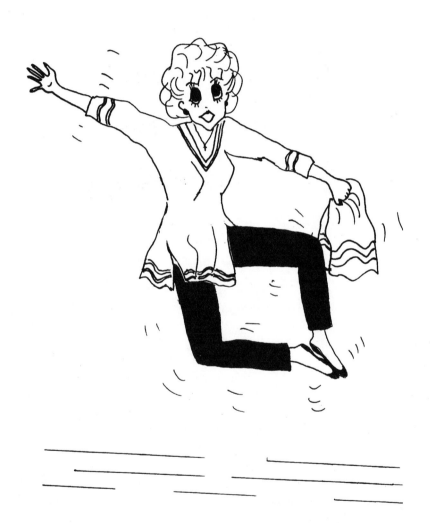

Chapter Six

My Answer: The Free TRAM Flap

On December 17, Jerry and I met Gloris at Dr. Cooper's office, and I was surprised to see that Dee was working for him. Dee had worked for fifteen years as office manager for Dr. Balek, our family doctor. Gloris, Jerry, and I waited in the examining room for just a few minutes before Dr. Cooper came into the room. He was a man of about forty. I was struck right away by his graciousness toward me. He was a gentleman, kind, and very much aware of the anguish I felt.

I was a little nervous; he didn't let on what he was thinking during my examination. When he was done, he folded his arms, smiled at me, and said, "Sherry, you are about the best candidate for this surgery that I have ever seen!" *Wow!* Music to *my* ears! He explained, the reasons: the shape of my breast was ideal; I was a nonsmoker; my stomach muscles had already been stretched during my pregnancies; I was "young" (I *really* liked this guy!); and I had no scars from prior surgeries. I had a virgin abdomen, untouched by another doctor's scalpel! (With the exception of not smoking, these are not requirements, just the "ideal.")

He spent a lot of time with us, patiently explaining this procedure. TRAM is the acronym for Transverse Rectus Abdominis Musculocutaneous. What a mouthful! By my translation it means *breast!* As he continued to talk, I realized it also meant *tummy tuck,* and that's not a bad thing!

The procedure Dr. Cooper and I decided on is called a Free TRAM Flap. It is a surgical procedure in which transverse (side to side) skin and fat, along with some abdominal muscle tissue, is cut free from the body and is transplanted to the new location, thus the name *Free* TRAM Flap. A pair of blood vessels (artery and vein) that come with the lower abdomen tissue are reconnected to existing blood vessels in the underarm area. This is done while the surgeon looks through a floor-mounted microscope. He uses a needle barely visible to the naked eye, threaded with filament finer than human hair. The Free TRAM Flap requires that the plastic surgeon have additional training in microscopic vascular surgery.

He explained that there were also other ways to accomplish autogenous tissue breast reconstruction. Autogenous means "from one's own body." One method is the Conventional TRAM Flap, which is similar to the Free TRAM Flap. It receives its blood supply through a tunnel created between the mastectomy site and the lower abdomen. The length of the surgery and recovery times for the Conventional and Free TRAM Flaps are much the same. The surgery usually takes five to eight hours, and the patient remains in the hospital two to five nights after the surgery. Although the patient is usually capable of self-care when discharged, total recovery from this surgery takes one to two months.

In some cases, hip or buttock tissue can be used as donor tissue for reconstructing a new breast. These procedures, however, are more difficult and involved, and since recovery time is longer, they are only done if the patient, for whatever reason, is not a candidate for either of the TRAM Flaps. Fortunately, I was a perfect candidate for the Free TRAM Flap!

Any of these procedures can be done years after the mastectomy. Even so, there are advantages to having reconstruction done in the same surgical procedure as the mastectomy. The general surgeon and the plastic surgeon can work as a team to get the best results cosmetically, and the plastic surgeon can use the breast that the general surgeon has removed as a pattern, enabling a more precise shape. It's ideal for the patient as well, because she doesn't have to deal with the vacancy on her chest.

After Dr. Cooper explained everything, he said with an apologetic tone, "We plastic surgeons like to have before and after pictures." As I posed for these mug shots, minus the mug, I told him, "My mother told me not to ever do this kind of thing!" He assured me that my anonymity would be protected. I was relieved to hear that my photos wouldn't show up in a magazine somewhere with a staple in my navel. There probably wasn't a big demand for women in their forties with poochy tummies anyway—but I thought it would be good to ask.

We scheduled my surgery for January 9, just three weeks away. I wanted to wait until after the holidays and our wedding anniversary, but to have it performed before Michael had to return to college. My doctors assured me that three weeks wouldn't endanger my health, since my cancer was slow growing and in the early stages.

As we left the office, I asked Gloris for her opinion of both Dr. Cooper and the procedure. She said she was impressed for the same reasons I was. She also said, "He commented that he loved doing this surgery, and when a doc loves doing a surgery that means he's good at it!" (That makes sense. You sure wouldn't love doing something you were bad at!) Gloris said, "Sherry, if I were where you are now, I would go for it!"

Jerry and I thanked Gloris for taking the time to meet us there. She said it was wonderful information for her to know and pass on to the surgeon she worked for.

Jerry was also impressed but didn't want to influence me one way or the other. He didn't want me to do this for him. If I was going to do it, it had to be for me. He assured me again that even if I didn't have any reconstruction he would lovingly support me. He just wanted me cancer free.

Since the time we were newlyweds a phrase from a Browning poem has always been precious to us, "Grow old along with me! The best is yet to be . . . ." I had it inscribed on Jerry's watch and painted on a plaque that hangs in our bedroom. That phrase remains the deep desire of our hearts. My "cancer experience" was the first time that our dream had ever been threatened.

Once I was home—and alone—I had some time to process it all and reflect on my appointment. I felt the most encouraged since this nightmare began. I thought, *I believe it's going to be okay. It will be traumatic, and I will have my ups and downs, but I now feel I can live with the results.*

I called my friends. They were relieved and happy for me, and out of the kindness of their hearts they even offered to donate their own tummy fat. Fortunately, I had enough of my own. Funny, I had never before been thankful for my poochy tummy. Bless those sons of mine for stretching out my once flat stomach! Lynn says that your stomach muscles come out with the placenta when you give birth, along with part of your brains. I believe her because I love her, and besides, it seems perfectly logical to me. At least it's a good excuse! I'm surprised the medical community hasn't picked up on it!

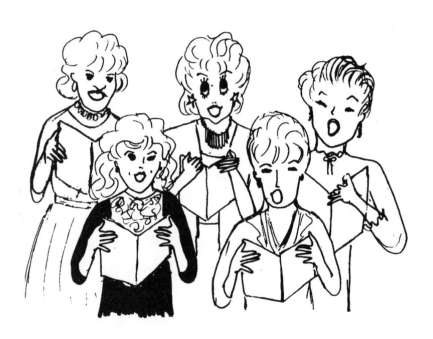

Chapter Seven
Choir Practice and Friendship

Christmas was only a week away, and we all tried our best to keep up our spirits. We went to David's basketball games, which meant more to us than they ever had before. Those games were some of the highlights in our lives at that point.

Another highlight in my life was being in the choir at our church. We had our Christmas cantata during that time, and it was wonderful. There are so many musically talented people at our church. I love being in our choir, even though my voice is just average. I used to say that my voice was mellow, that is until I learned that mellow meant overripe and very nearly rotten! Now I say it's an average voice.

I am no great asset to either the choir or the music ministry of our church. The choir, however, is an enormous asset to me. Pastor Rich and Marge are a team, not only in marriage but in his ministry as well. Marge is such a gifted pianist, and in my opinion, is the ultimate woman. She is kind, gracious, loving, very unassuming, and she's a true blessing to her husband, children, and everyone who knows her. Pastor Rich, I'm sure, knows that I am no Sandi Patti or Barbra Streisand; but he still allows me to come to choir and even tells me that I'm missed when I'm not there. However, he does make me stand in the back row! He says it's because I'm tall, but I think it's because the microphones are in the front. He doesn't want me to scare the congregation, especially the first-time visitors! Our church service is broadcast on the radio—I think that also influences him.

Practice is wonderful on Wednesday nights. We sing together, laugh, cry, and pray together. It's like a very big extended family.

I remember one night that seemed like it was out of an old *I Love Lucy* episode. I arrived at practice a little late, and the only seat available was in the middle of the second row. The choir chairs are set up in rows, each row graduating about six inches higher than the previous one. It was winter, I had on a heavy coat, and my arms were full of music books. The choir was already in the process of practicing a song, so I was trying to sneak in as quietly as possible. I excused myself as I made my way to the only empty seat in the soprano section. Unfortunately, I stepped on one of my fellow sopranos' tender feet. As she cried out in pain, and I swung around to quietly whisper an apology to her, my purse (a shoulder bag) fell off my shoulder and crashed down on top of the head of an unsuspecting gal in the front row. Her hand automatically flew to the top of her head as she shrieked in pain. I turned my attention to her, intending to grovel for forgiveness. I looked up at Rich and noticed no one was singing and all eyes were on me. Rich was standing there with his arms folded, tapping his foot and looking terribly stern. Apparently, they had all noticed my grand and graceful entrance. I grinned a sheepish grin at Rich and said, "Sorry."

Rich said, "If you could *just* come in and take a seat like *normal* people!" We all laughed as I took my seat. I took off my coat, got out my book, looked up at Rich, and noticed that everyone was watching me. Rich said he wanted to make sure I was ready before attempting the song again. How thoughtful!

Rich always says that I am his favorite person in the world to tease, and I love to give it back to him! He has always been thrilled that I am eight months older than he is and believes that it is his mission in life to inform the general population of this news, telling them to closely check me out for wrinkles. He really *looks* gobs older than I do, and I feel that it is my duty to point that out to him. This dialogue has become quite a routine.

He thinks, and likes to share with anyone who will listen, that I am "Wacko" because my hair is red. I, at least, *have* hair and feel the need to point that out to him—in love, of course! He tells me it's better to have no hair than red hair. I think not!

For weeks leading up to Rich's 40th birthday, I bought the worst cards I could find that described the negative attributes of growing older. I signed them "The Red Phantom" and left them in his box at the church. One day I left a bumper sticker that said, "Tease me about my age and I'll beat you with my cane!" This sort of backfired on me. The following Sunday, while the rest of us were in Sunday School (where we were supposed to be), Richie Ray was lurking out in the parking lot, searching for my car. He found it and put that nasty bumper sticker on *my* bumper! I guess he figured out who "The Red Phantom" was.

All of this teasing is done with much love and all in fun and has been going on since Richie Ray had hair. It's not that Rich has no hair, it's just that it's not as evenly distributed as it used to be!

As a choir we do have a lot of fun, and we really do love each other. I believe the choir, under Rich's direction, truly practices what we are instructed in Romans 12:15, "When others are happy, be happy with them. If they are sad, share in their sorrow" (LB). I believe that they genuinely shared in my sorrow. I received many phone calls, cards, and hugs from those special people. They even wept with me when I wept. I felt the most warmth when they prayed with me, particularly when we broke up into our sections and the sopranos prayed together. I knew that those women loved me and felt my sorrow; and when I found out about the TRAM Flap reconstruction, they rejoiced with me. That's what it's all about. Jesus instructed us to love one another, and I believe that the choir at my church obeys these instructions.

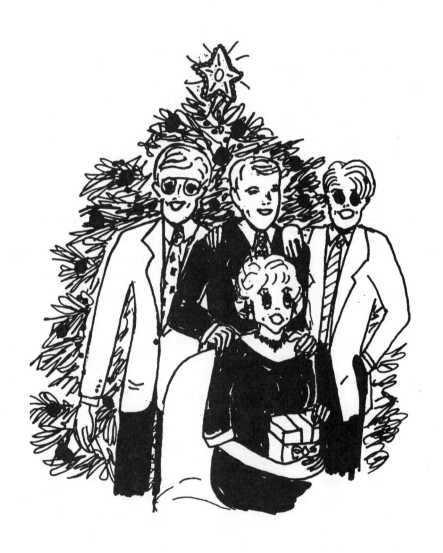

Chapter Eight
It Won't Be a Blue Christmas!

Monday, December 24, 1990
"Dear Lord,

It's Christmas Eve. The candlelight service at church was beautiful. Ronnie sang "Bethlehem Morning," as only she can. It was exquisite. I can't help wondering if it's the last time I will hear her sing it here on earth.

As the surgery gets closer, it feels like someone is squeezing my heart. Is there something wrong with my heart, or is it anxiety? I have never had surgery before, and this seems like a really big one to start out with! Cancer, amputation, several hours of reconstruction—it all seems so overwhelming.

I have come to the conclusion that my heart is fine, that fear is what is squeezing my heart. Even so, at night when it's dark and still, my imagination runs rampant. I wonder if something will happen to me during the surgery, if my heart, exhausted from being in the clutches of fear, will stop on the operating table. I know, Lord, that there are worse ways of dying. If I were to die in surgery, I will have told my family how much I love them. There would be no pain involved. I would just go peacefully to sleep and awaken in your presence, Lord. I will get to see my beloved grandmother, Nana, again. I will be in a place where there is no cancer, no evil, no sadness, no tears. But Lord, I am just not ready yet. I grieve at the thought of leaving my family of men.

Jerry broke down and cried tonight. I am so glad he finally let it out. He has been so strong for me. I adore him with everything in me. We have been together for over half of our lives, and I believe that we are more in love than when we took our vows. I know that he is a gift from you Lord. Thank you! I also thank you, Lord, for Michael and David, so precious, indeed, to me. It feels as if they are my heart walking around outside of my body, each one completely unique, each one so loved by their mother. Even in this situation I am truly blessed. Happy Birthday, Jesus!"

Christmas morning was fun! We had Christmas music on the stereo, presents, and "twisty-tails" (sweet rolls), which have become a Christmas tradition. Every year I tell my family, "Maybe I won't make twisty-tails this year. All that sugar really isn't that good for us; we really don't need them, do we?" Then I stand back and watch my three guys, each one more than six feet tall, whine and beg. I let them think they talked me into it one more year—of course, in reality, I would never deprive them of twisty-tails on Christmas morning.

Things have certainly changed around here! I remember when the boys would jump on our bed at 4:00 A.M., excited beyond words. We would plead with them to go back to bed until 6:00, and bribe them by telling them they could take their stockings back to their room and play quietly.

This year as Jerry and I cuddled on the couch with our coffee, we listened to Christmas music and admired our tree. It was decorated with such care, most of the ornaments homemade, each having a special memory.

We finally woke up the boys, because *we* were the ones excited and wanting to dig into the gifts. Things have definitely changed around here. We do get to sleep longer, but I miss those two little boys running through the house giggling as they bring us our stockings in bed, begging us to get up so they can attack the packages under the tree. I guess when you are in high school and college you are too cool to get excited on Christmas morning. I, however, am *never* too cool to get excited about presents. In fact, *gift* is one of my favorite four letter words!

We had our family Christmas at home and then spent the afternoon with Pastor Rich and Marge and their family, and Dr. Phil and Jan and their family at Phil and Jan's house. We snacked until dinner, ate until we were about to pop, then had a brief time-out before dessert. I must confess that it was kind of nice to eat whatever and however much I wanted. I joked about my great excuse for "porking out": I had to make sure I had enough tummy for my new breast, after all! I told Marge I was eating for medicinal purposes. She poked my tummy and said, "It's coming along!"

At home that evening, Jerry and I cuddled in each other's arms as we fell asleep. I silently asked the Lord if cancer would be a threat to future Christmases with my three men. "I feel so safe when Jerry holds me. How could something be a threat to my life when I'm feeling so loved and protected? Maybe this is all just a bad dream that will be over in the morning. Is that possible, Lord?"

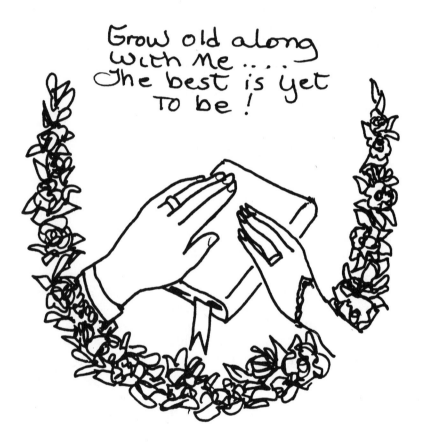

Chapter Nine

Twenty-two Years: Our Wedding Anniversary

Friday, December 28, 1990
"Dear Lord,

December 28, 1990—it's our wedding anniversary. Jerry brought me a beautiful coral rose, wrote an even more beautiful note, then took me to the Mustard Seed, one of our favorite restaurants.

It's hard to believe we have been married for twenty-two years. That is half of our lives! We have grown closer over the years. I believe I love him more fervently than when we were married in Hayward, California, more than two decades ago.

There seems to be such an urgency to express our love to each another. Cancer can do that to you. Every moment with someone you love is precious; you savor every second on the clock. *Is this our last anniversary, Lord? Please, don't let it be so! Help me to trust you. Lord, calm my heart! Thank you for the gift of twenty-two years in a loving marriage!*"

A Bit of History

Nothing like cancer to make an anniversary stand out in your mind! It's a long time, twenty-two years. Jerry has laugh lines by those wonderful blue eyes now, and his hair is more gray than brown. Even so, my heart still jumps like it did April 1, 1968, when I first laid eyes on him. April Fool's Day . . . he's still waiting for the joke to be over! He tells me he could never divorce me on grounds of boredom. I *choose* to take that as a compliment!

Jerry was a Navy corpsman, a medic, at the old Oak Knoll Naval Hospital in Oakland, California. Though in the process of building a new facility, they were still in the old barracks-style hospital. It was during the war in Vietnam. Injured men were first taken to a hospital in Okinawa, Japan, then flown to a stateside hospital before going home. Oak Knoll was one such hospital on the West Coast.

Coming of age in the sixties was interesting, both exciting and unsettling. We were children in the fifties when our country was at peace. Life seemed simple then, even if your family wasn't an Ozzie and Harriet, June Cleaver, or Donna Reed type family. (Did those women really clean toilets in a dress and 4-inch heels?) There was still a kind of innocence, a faith in God and country. Then, when we were teenagers in the middle and late sixties, our country was suddenly in turmoil, and there were rumors that God was "dead." Racial tension and war protests brought on riots. Leaders were being gunned down, and we were seeing it firsthand on TV in our living rooms. It wasn't a movie; it was real—and it was happening in America, "the land of the free and home of the brave." We had always won wars because we were the "good guys," and good guys always win. It's a rule! Suddenly, we were the "bad guys," and people over thirty years old weren't to be trusted.

It was a strange setting in which to meet the love of your life and fall in love. Neither one of us was looking for Cupid to blast us with an arrow. Jerry was having fun as a bachelor, living off base in an apartment in Oakland with his friends and fellow corpsmen, Doug and Jon. I was going to a local college and living at home with my mother and stepfather, my brothers and sister. Weekends were fun with my girlfriends, and I was writing to a fellow who was stationed in Guam.

Jan had been a friend since high school. We were "hangin' out" at her house when she got a phone call from a distraught woman who was the mother of one of her former boyfriends. The woman's son had just been in a car accident. She lived several hours away and couldn't make the trip, so she was asking Jan to go visit him. He was in the Navy, so he had been taken to Oak Knoll Naval Hospital. Jan, not wanting to go to the hospital alone, asked me to accompany her. That's where I first saw Jerry, the corpsman taking care of him. He was wearing a white tech jacket that buttoned at the side of the neck, just like the one Dr. Ben Casey wore. We couldn't seem to take our eyes off of each other. They were like magnets being pulled together. We would sneak a peek at one another and quickly look away. (It was strange. Who can explain that amazing phenomenon we call chemistry? Either you got it, or you ain't! If I could somehow bottle and sell it, I would be a bazillionaire!)

I tried to tag along with Jan on most of her trips to the hospital. During one of those visits, we walked into the ward while Jerry was feeding a patient whose eyes were covered with bandages. The patient asked me if the sun was shining, and I told him it was. He said he was afraid that he would never see the sunlight again. As I stood at the foot of that man's bed, Jerry and I encouraged him, together. I think it was the first time we had actually spoken to one another, and even though our words were directed to Jerry's patient, our eyes were directed to each other. I was so touched by the compassionate way that he planted a seed of hope as he fed lunch to his patient.

Finally, he asked me out! We went to an Elvis movie on base, and it cost him an entire quarter! It was the first time I had watched an Elvis movie and not been totally captivated by Elvis. I just remember how thrilled I was to be sitting beside this handsome and strong yet compassionate man who didn't even try to hold my hand.

We spent a lot of time walking around the grounds at the hospital. We became friends, talking about everything, sharing our hopes and dreams. He told me about his family, his parents, and the Oregon ranch they bought when Jerry was in his teens. He shared with pride about his older brother, Ken, a commercial pilot who was about to be married, and about his sister, Jean, and her family in Portland. Jerry was the baby. I could almost envision the ranch next to the river, the wheat growing and swaying in the breeze, and the tall pine trees as he described them all to me. I tried to imagine him in the saddle, looking as dashing as Roy Rogers as he ran his horse, Reno, through that beautiful country.

He loved his family and I was afraid I was starting to love him. I had only been in love once before, with my high school sweetheart. When we broke up, I was heartbroken. I didn't know if I wanted to risk being hurt again. I shared my fear with a girlfriend, wondering if I should stop seeing him. She told me I was crazy and that I could be running away from the love of my life. She didn't begin to know the wisdom she exuded or how prophetic her words turned out to be.

In June, Jerry flew up to Washington to be in his brother's wedding. I was so lonely for him. Our relationship had advanced to handholding, and he hugged and kissed me before he left. But we hadn't spoken of love or any kind of commitment. All I knew was that every time he came near me, my heart would start pounding, my face would get hot, my hands would get clammy, and I would get weak in the knees. Those strange symptoms led me to determine that I was either wildly in love, or extremely allergic to him!

During the two weeks he was gone, I spent the days at school and the evenings at home. I was invited to San Francisco for dinner and a show on a blind date with a friend and her boyfriend. It sounded like a wonderful time, and my friend thought I was nuts for turning it down; but I just wanted to stay home and wait for Jerry to come back. I worked on my tan in the back yard. Before he left, Jerry and I had made a bet that whoever had the best tan when he returned would be taken for a steak dinner by the loser. . . . I won!

I waited patiently for him to return, only to have him tell me that he had taken an old girlfriend out while he was in Washington. My heart sank—until he told me he was miserable (*Good!*) and couldn't stop wishing he was with me. Being with her made him realize that he was in love with me and didn't want to be with anyone else. I was thrilled but managed to "maintain my cool" on the outside. I silently thought it would be a nice gesture to write that dear girl a thank you note!

Our courtship was a bittersweet time for us because the military patients continued to touch our hearts. We were only twenty-one years old, but many of the injured men were even younger. Several of the men were amputees. Some of the patients had lost their sight and still had shrapnel scars on their faces. Some had broken spirits. But most spirits were strong. I remember overhearing two men, both double leg amputees, sitting in their wheelchairs having a friendly argument about which branch of the armed forces was the best. I didn't hear the end of the argument, but each passionately loved his branch and argued with such spirit, such pride!

During Jerry's and my courtship, John Filippelli, a friend of mine from high school, was killed in Vietnam. He was hit by ground fire while on a helicopter search mission. He was only twenty-one years old, and he was the first friend my own age that I had ever lost to death. My last conversation with John was in the college library. He had decided to buckle down and put more effort into his classes; his other option was being drafted and going to Vietnam. The next thing I heard, he was on his way to Vietnam. He was there nine months, and then, he was gone.

It was hard to believe; he had been tall and strong, a football player with a dazzling smile who looked like he could conquer the world.

John's death was devastating to me, not only because he was my friend, but because the Navy could decide they wanted Jerry over there at any time. As terrible as it was to lose my young friend, the thought that I could lose Jerry was horrifying.

An interesting era it was to court and fall in love. Probably much like when the generation prior to ours sent their men off to war during WWII, but with the difference that then there was patriotism in the air. We were the heroes then; the country was behind the war. This time we wanted to believe we were in a "John Wayne war" that was necessary and right, but there were loud and angry protests saying it was wrong. Was it possible that my friend John was killed for no reason, like the irate protesters were saying? I wasn't particularly politically minded, just young and in love and shaken by the unrest in our country.

Jerry had met my family and they loved him. In September, we were on our way to Oregon so that I could meet his family. The country was every bit as beautiful as I had imagined. Troy, Oregon, was small (population twenty-two) and isolated. It takes two hours of driving beside the winding Grande Ronde River to get to the nearest town. I was a city slicker who had never before seen country like Troy, Oregon, or the road to it! I was convinced that if I sat too close to the passenger side of the car, I would cause the car to plummet over the edge and into the canyon—and we would be forever lost to our families and the world!

I had never tasted corn as sweet as the corn Jerry's mother grew, nor had I ever met a cow personally that would soon be dinner! Jerry's dad, as I was about to take a bite of steak, would wink at me and say, "Remember ole Bessie's big brown eyes? I think ole Bessie really liked you." I preferred to think that beef floated down from heaven, wrapped ever so neatly in cellophane, and landed in the meat case at the local market. I would rather not have known that there was blood involved. However, I surmised that if I was going to marry the son of a rancher, it was time to face the filet of facts, the reality of rump roast.

What an eventful time we had! I forded the river in a flatbed truck with Jerry's dad. (I was either nuts or trying to prove I wasn't a sissy!) Later, Jerry and I enjoyed one of the crisp autumn afternoons on horseback. I rode Jerry's mother's horse, Taco. Taco was an interesting critter who, after eating, would walk over to a fence post, hook his front teeth to the post, and then burp—loudly.

When asked if I wanted to ride Scotty, the donkey, I readily agreed. After climbing onto Scotty's back, Jerry's dad informed me that when Scotty had a stranger on his back, he would take off running like his tail was on fire, come to a dead stop, put his head down, and his passenger would tumble over the top of his head to the ground. The look on my face, after hearing this little donkey quirk, sent them into hysterics. It seemed a little strange to me, of course, but Scotty was the first donkey I had ever met, so what did I have to compare him to? Luckily for me, Scotty decided to control his sudden burst of energy. This was a ranch, however, and I have always suspected that there was a little bull being thrown around in honor of the greenhorn.

I even saw my first rattlesnake, which had ferocious fangs, and I'm positive, was about 57 feet long, at the very least! That first visit to the ranch was quite an experience for a wimpy city slicker, such as I.

Before we left for home, Jerry's dad gave him one of Jerry's mother's diamonds to have made into a ring for me. We hadn't yet set the date but were certain we wanted to spend our lives together. And although we have had our share of challenges, we have always been confident that we made the right choice.

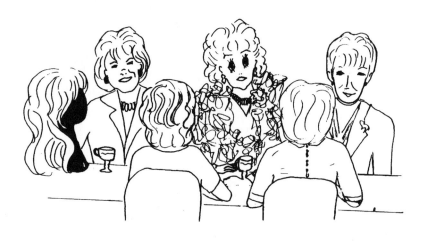

Chapter Ten

The God-Is-Faithful Luncheon

On January 3, Ronnie, Peggy, and Keegan wanted to take me to lunch. My surgery was less than a week away, and the dread I felt was a heavy weight dragging me down. They wanted to show me their love and encouragement, but I just wanted to stay home in my sweats, my hair pulled back in a rubber band, the blinds closed. I called Ronnie, who had planned our lunch, and tried to make my excuses. She said they were all looking forward to it and I wasn't going to be a "nerd" and back out. Determination is Ronnie's middle name, and I knew it was futile to argue with her. Besides, I didn't want to disappoint them so I reluctantly consented.

I had to literally drag my reluctant, lethargic fanny to the mirror and slap a little makeup on my face in an attempt to look and feel alive. It's ironic. Lynn and I joke that *lunch* is our life. That day I felt as if I were being hauled to the gallows rather than to lunch with three dear friends from the choir.

They picked me up, and as Peggy drove us downtown, Ronnie turned around from the front seat and presented me with a tape. She slipped it into the cassette player, and the song that started to play was called, "He's Been Faithful," performed by the incredible Damaris Carbaugh. It was clear that this song had profound meaning to her, and it was a special gift of love from her heart to mine. I thanked her, but all I felt in my heart was an overwhelming sadness. As tears started to roll down my cheeks, Keegan, seated next to me, reached over and held my hand.

Located in downtown Spokane is an actual old flourmill that was redone into, among other things, quaint little boutiques, shops, and restaurants, one of which was our lunch destination, Clinkerdaggers. We browsed for a while in one of the boutiques, then headed for the restaurant. Escorted to our table, I was astounded to discover that it was filled with my friends: Judy, Marge, Marcia, Jan, Lynn, Donna, and now Ronnie, Peggy, and Keegan. They had reserved a spot for me in the center. As I was getting over the shock, they pinned a beautiful corsage on my sweater and presented me with a gift, a guest book. On the first page of the guest book was written, "The God-Is-Faithful Luncheon, in Honor of Sherry Lynn." Inside the guest book, each one of them had expressed their love to me, along with words of encouragement and scripture. Ronnie said I was to take the book to the hospital for visitors to sign, and she would invite people who came during my surgery to sign it so I would know who had been there.

Lynn brought a special "hospital ensemble" for me to wear. It started with a truly *ugly* hot pink nightgown and a trashy feather boa. She said, "I know that hot pink clashes with your hair, but never fear, for I have solved that problem!" Then she pulled out a very bouffant, very long, platinum blonde wig. (I think I saw it on a hooker as we drove to the restaurant. I couldn't believe my friend Lynn accosted a hooker and stole her hair!) Next, she presented me with a pair of very feminine and stylish cow slippers, enhanced by their little tongues hanging out on the floor. A wonderful ensemble! The other patients would have been green . . . err . . . hot pink with envy! *Of course, if I had chosen to wear this lovely ensemble at the hospital, the staff might have insisted that I add one of their "captivating" white jackets. (You know, the one that wraps your arms snugly around your waist and ties in the back!)* My delightful friends plopped the wig on top of my head, held the less than lovely nightie up to me, wrapped the feather boa around my neck, and took pictures. I'm quite sure I was stunning—I know I was stunned.

We laughed throughout the luncheon. The servers at the restaurant as well as the diners at surrounding tables got into the act, offering to take the pictures for us, laughing, and admiring my outfit. A group of businessmen stopped by our table on their way out. One of them put his hand on my shoulder and told me he had been watching our party and couldn't figure out if my friends *really* liked me or *really* hated me! Then he smiled, winked, patted my shoulder, and said, "Nice outfit!"

Those around us, affected by our luncheon, probably thought it was my birthday. I'm sure they would have been shocked if they had known that I had cancer and that my friends wanted to brighten my day with an encouragement luncheon!

We had a wonderful luncheon, and I basked in the love and support that was poured out so abundantly on me on a day that had started out so low. Thanks to those dear ladies, I'm still affected by the memory of it. What a wonderful way to have given joy to someone whose joy tank was seriously below empty. Their gift of that wonderful afternoon filled my tank to overflowing. I have been truly blessed with amazing friends who not only laughed with me but who were willing also to cry with me and share my pain. The Lord used them to, " . . . turn my mourning into dancing" (Psalm 30:11, KJV). When I left the restaurant, my heart was dancing from the warmth of their love.

When Jerry came home from work, I was wearing the ensemble, wig and all, for the full effect. He commented again on how life with me is never boring. He, too, was touched and very grateful for the gift of love and encouragement that was given to me on that snowy afternoon at Clinkerdagger's restaurant.

That evening we went to David's basketball game. It was intense, but David's team, the Eagles, won!

I thanked the Lord that night for the way He turned a melancholy morning into a heartwarming afternoon of affection and affirmation. What a wonderful way to be reminded that we have the ability and the privilege to lift someone up, share their burden, and plant a bit of joy into their heavy hearts. Their compassion and thoughtfulness not only ministered to me but affected those around us. It was a contagious afternoon. Those people in the restaurant were aware that there was something special about that luncheon, and they wanted to be a part of it. They never knew that on that afternoon the Lord used His people to lance the boil of fear and dread, extract some of the poison, and replace it with the healing balm of joy. They never knew what they had witnessed was a "divine" lunch date: "The God-Is-Faithful Luncheon."

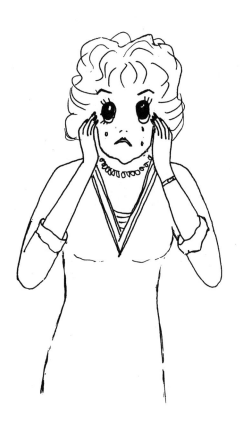

Chapter Eleven
Tears and Fears

It was Sunday, and my surgery was only three days away. I was in the choir singing praise songs when tears started to silently pour down my cheeks. I really don't know the reason for the tears. It may have been the praise songs we were singing, or perhaps it was just looking at the congregation, the many faces that were so very dear to me. I was humiliated and embarrassed by my lack of control and didn't know what to do. If I left, I would draw more attention to myself, and that was the last thing I wanted. I wished that there was some magical way I could just disappear!

I couldn't seem to make the tears stop, and I wondered why God put tear ducts where they were so noticeable. How humiliating it was to be in front of a church full of people and not be able to manage my emotions! If I were God, I would have taken a person's pride into consideration before placing tear ducts in such a conspicuous place! Under the fingernails would have been my choice; then, if the dam burst and you didn't want anyone to see you cry, you could simply slip your hands into your pockets, and your tears would disappear!

I hoped and prayed that no one noticed, that I would be spared that indignity. As I looked down, however, I saw Marcia crying and Brent trying to console her. Linda had her head bowed, and knowing her heart, I am confident that she was praying for me, asking God to give me strength and courage.

I was relieved and grateful when the singing was finally over so I could escape and my fear and dread would not be on display. I quickly went downstairs and got out of my choir robe, uncharacteristically avoiding eye contact with my fellow choir members. I rushed through the basement and up the stairs to the back of the church. Having chosen the last pew, I sat close to the door to be able to leave quickly, unnoticed. Jerry finished his ushering duties and took his seat beside me. I held on tightly to his hand, praying earnestly that Pastor Tom's sermon would be short and sweet. I wanted so desperately to run home and hide. I thought that if he would just put his sermon on fast-forward, I could flee and possibly manage to salvage at least a molecule of self-respect. Safe at home, no one could see how weak I felt. I was embarrassed by my lack of faith and trust in the Lord and could think of fifty women in the church who could face this ordeal with dignity, women who would glorify the Lord with the peace that surpasses all understanding that Philippians 4:7 talks about. Where was *my* piece of that peace? I felt like a sniveling coward who had disgraced the Lord in her weakness . . . ashamed . . . a failure in my faith.

At the end of the service, I jumped up and headed for the door, trying desperately to make a quick exit. But suddenly I was totally surrounded by countless women in the church. My faithful friend Donna was standing by my side and was as overwhelmed as I when each woman, young and old, hugged me and told me she could imagine how I felt. Individually, they expressed their love for me and promised that I would be in their prayers. They assured me that the Lord loved me immensely and would send His angels to assist the doctors in my surgery. I felt that these dear ladies were angels themselves whom God was using to show me that He doesn't expect us to always be strong. He wants us just to be real so that others may have the joy of ministering to us and we can receive comfort from them.

God is *always* there for us, but we can't touch Him or see Him, so sometimes we need someone with skin on who can hug us and wipe away our tears. If, in our pride, we refuse to be transparent, if we always wear our phony, "I've got everything under control" masks, we cheat ourselves out of the love we can receive from Him through each other. The Lord loves us individually, and very often He chooses to demonstrate that love to us through one another. He knows that sometimes we need to *feel* the hugs and *hear* those words of encouragement. After all, it's no secret to Him. He made us that way.

So, God, I guess it's okay that you put our tear ducts in our eyes, right on our faces, above our noses for everyone to see. If you had put them under our fingernails, as *I* proposed, the possibility of another paralyzing predicament could pop up. For then, if we cried hard and put our hands in our pockets to hide the tears, it might look as if we had wet our pants! It's just possible that this would be even more humiliating! Lord, I guess you know best after all.

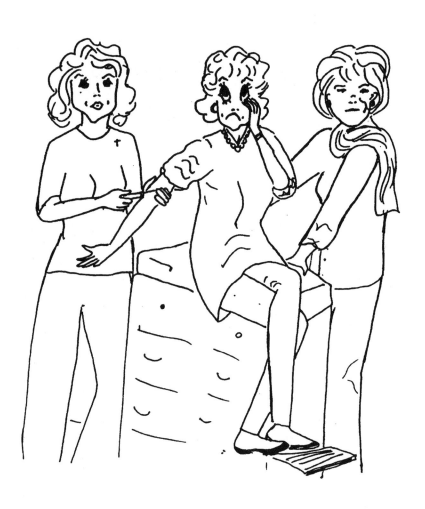

Chapter Twelve

Pre-Surgery Jitters

On Monday, January 7, it was too real, too close. The hands on the clock were moving too fast. If it had been possible, I think I would have gone to the clock on the wall, opened the little door, and stopped the pendulum—or at least slowed it down. I wasn't ready yet! But then, is anyone ever ready to have cancer, to experience the trauma of having part of their body amputated, part of their femininity heartlessly stolen by a vicious disease?

Lynn took me to lunch, to see Dr. Cooper, then to register and do the blood work at the hospital. It was snowing, big time, so the ride downtown was exciting to say the least! I wasn't worried though. I figured if I got killed in the snowstorm, I would have a good excuse for not showing up for surgery. Since I was considering not showing up anyway, this way my truancy would be excused. I can see it now. Jerry could have written a note:

> *Please excuse my Sherry's absence under your knife. She was called out of town—to heaven, to be exact. She had to help her Father. He wanted to consult with her about a little matter of relocating tear ducts.*

An excused absence would have been great, but since I didn't go to heaven, I had to show up for surgery.

Of course, before surgery you must participate in that wonderful tradition called "Pre-surgery Registration." Doctors and hospitals can get quite persnickety if you don't show up for their pre-surgery stuff. And since it's definitely not wise to irritate someone who has you drugged *and* is holding a knife over your naked body, it's advisable to be a cooperative and well-behaved patient—well, at least cooperative!

In order to psych ourselves up for that undertaking, lunch was strategically placed *first* on our agenda. Doctors and hospitals are not our forte, but we *are* extremely gifted at "doing lunch."

Lynnie and I can usually squeeze a little humor out of just about any calamity. That day, however, we were a little more solemn than usual. Lynn, trying to comfort me, looked at me with loving concern and said, "Sherry, I hate that you have to go through this! But, it's through these kinds of painful experiences that we gain great depth."

I replied, "But, Lynn, you don't understand. I *like* being shallow! I didn't sign up anywhere to be a woman of great depth. I'm very comfortable with shallow—it works for me!" Lynn nearly fell off her chair howling with laughter. The more she laughed, the more I laughed. We laughed because it was truth.

We'd all love to be people of great wisdom and profundity, but not if it causes us pain. However, just as we had physical growing pains as children, we experience emotional growing pains all through our lives.

I know that when I see the battle of a trial marching toward me, I tend to jump into the first available foxhole, cover my eyes in denial, and cry out to God to take it away. Being of sanguine temperament, I am *not* a willing participant unless an experience is at least a little bit fun. I wanted to say to God, "Sorry, I don't *do* cancer. Try someone strong and spiritually worthy of this immense trial. If you need someone to do, say, a mild flu—you have your warrior! Even though throwing up is grossly

88

unladylike, I would be willing to sacrifice and sign up for flu. But I don't like the idea of signing up for cancer!"

Donna says, "We are all changing, growing, and becoming all that God created us to be!" It's a process, it takes time, and often we must endure great pain and suffering along the way. The blessings usually come *after* the battle. The battle is the tough part! If we can struggle through the battle with the strength of the Lord and survive in spite of our battle scars, we have a victory!

Sometimes a person fighting a disease like cancer needs a transfusion. In my fight, I didn't need a physical transfusion, I needed a spiritual one! I was so weary at times that I couldn't even ask God for His strength to sustain me. That's when my faithful friends and family stood in the gap and cried out to God on my behalf.

Hopefully, with God's help, there will be a day when I won't be a wimpy warrior. I trust that I am, "changing, growing, and becoming all I was meant to be." I will have arrived completely only when I am in the presence of the Lord.

The crime is not that a person hasn't arrived, but that he or she would refuse to start the journey. The crime is lying to oneself, thinking one has it all together with nothing to learn. How arrogant, how frightening, how foolish!

Trials develop perseverance. In my opinion, it would be so difficult to persevere without the grace of God. Romans 5:3–5 says, ". . . we must rejoice in our sufferings, because we know that suffering produces perseverance; perseverance character; and character, hope. And hope does not disappoint us, because God has poured out His love into our hearts by the Holy Spirit whom He has given us."

Notice that it says "rejoice *in* our sufferings," not *for* our sufferings. I don't care how spiritual and strong I am feeling on any particular day, I couldn't see myself saying to God, "Lord, I want to rejoice in the privilege of having cancer!" Maybe there are people who can *sincerely* do that—not me! I can (and did) say, however, "Lord, I want to rejoice that I am yours, and because of that relationship, I know you have my best interest at heart. I can't imagine how this can be for my best interest, but I trust that you know what you're doing in allowing this in my life. I *do* rejoice that my cancer is in the beginning stages. I *do* rejoice in the people you have placed around me to love and encourage me. I *do* rejoice that Dr. Cooper recently moved into town and that I am an excellent candidate for this reconstruction. I *do* thank you that the wonderful skill you gifted to him will enable me to feel whole after this cruel surgery. I *do* rejoice that you comfort me with your love letter, the Bible. I *do* rejoice that when this is all over you will use it somehow for my good and your glory."

At my appointment with Dr. Cooper, I was to give him a medical history and have him answer any questions that I might have regarding my surgery. I was having a fairly colossal case of pre-surgery jitters, so I asked Dr. Cooper if I was doing the right thing. I'd had a couple of conversations where people had tried to talk me into having just the mastectomy and not the reconstruction I had chosen. They felt it was "too big a surgery" or "too long to be under the anesthetic." When I asked Dr. Cooper about these concerns, he put my mind at ease. When he addressed the length of time under the anesthetic, he explained that it was much like flying an airplane: it's the takeoff and landing that are crucial, not so much the time in the air.

As for the complexity of the surgery, I was "young," and apart from the cancer, I was healthy; he didn't foresee any problems. As we talked, my confidence in my choice of reconstruction grew strong again. After all, women have "tummy tucks" every day for cosmetic reasons, and the excess muscle, skin, and fat are discarded. In my case, they would be recycled, so to speak, used to rebuild an absent breast. I would leave the hospital with my body somewhat intact. I felt the psychological benefits outweighed any concerns.

Dr. Cooper had tried to locate some of his former TRAM Flap patients for me. It would have been helpful to have talked to someone who had chosen this surgery as a form of reconstruction. Unfortunately, military people are not known for nesting in one location for long periods of time, so he could find no one. To hear a woman say, "I chose the TRAM Flap and am thrilled with the results," to detect a smile in her voice as I heard encouraging words, would have been worth everything to me at that point.

Dr. Cooper assured me that no one on whom he had done the TRAM Flap had ever expressed regret to him regarding their choice. He said that my second thoughts at that point were understandable and quite normal, and assured me that I was a perfect candidate for the reconstructive surgery. Although he was very reassuring, he took care not to influence my decision, gently reminding me that it was a very personal decision that only I could make.

As my appointment drew to a close, Dr. Cooper asked me if there was anything else he could do for me. I started to cry and said, "If only you could make my cancer disappear, so I wouldn't have to go through this!"

"I wish I could do that for you," he said sadly, and I believe he meant it.

I was given my paperwork to take to the hospital, our next stop. I had only been a patient in the hospital three times: once to be born and twice to give birth. The first time, I don't quite remember. The second and third times didn't start out to be much fun, but the immeasurable joy I felt when my baby boys were placed in my arms made me forget the lack of fun I experienced on arrival. This time, instead of going into the hospital to be presented with a precious gift from my body, I felt that I was being forced to go to a cruel place that was going to steal a precious part of my body.

At the hospital, Lynn and I managed to get me registered. That seemed to go well, until that nice, unsuspecting lady wanted to draw blood out of my arm. It wouldn't have bothered me so much if she hadn't insisted on involving a needle, a needle that looked at least nine (and three quarters) feet long. If modern science would come up with a way to draw blood without involving a needle, Sherry Lynn, and a whole buncha' five- and six-year-olds, would be a lot less fussy about it! I kinda suspect that needles are even against my religion. In the whole Bible, a needle is only mentioned once, and that involved a camel—not a fraidy cat!

Lynn and I tried to trick her into forgetting her sinister deed. We involved her in a clever conversation that would have confused anyone. We talked about how often we shave our legs. I do it every other day. Lynn does it every other month, whether they need it or not! (Just kidding Lynnie.) I have somewhat forgotten how it came up. I think I was worried about having gorilla legs in the hospital. We decided that by the time I cared whether my legs were smooth and hairless or not, I would probably feel up to shaving them.

Alas, our trickery didn't work. She was too shrewd for us. She insisted on drawing my blood. I had to at least fake the demeanor of a mature adult. *This will require an Academy Award performance!*, I thought. She, of course, couldn't get my wimpy vein on the first try, which made me tense and her megatense. After a couple of tries she succeeded, pulled the needle out, and said, "I need a drink!" We all laughed about my wimpy veins and how thankful we were that this nasty, bloodsucking procedure was over.

Just then the phone rang. She answered it and quickly showed the same look of terror that a soldier returning to the front lines might have. "Really?" she asked. "Are you sure? Okay." She hung up, took a deep breath, and said, "They want another tube of blood."

I said, "What is this, a vampire deli?" Now, Lynn and I had to calm the technician and reassure her that it would be all right. Luckily, she was successful on the first try. It was just possible that she was more thrilled than even I. (Lynn and I have a horrible feeling that she picked up the phone to quit her job just after we walked out the door.)

Tuesday, January 8, 1990
"Dear Lord,
 The surgery is tomorrow, and I've been uptight all day. I wish
that invisible stress monster would quit squeezing my heart, or
would at least loosen its grip. I try to remind myself that each
step I take closer to this surgery takes me closer to the time that
I will be walking with it behind me. I *long* to have this dreadful
experience behind me. The wisdom and perspective that comes
after a trial seems so far away. If only I could "fast forward,"
reflect on this nightmare, and skip the experience.
 I've kept busy cleaning house, doing laundry, and baking so
my men will have goodies in my absence. Lots of phone calls
and well wishes today: Mom, Dad, Jerry's dad, and Claudia called
from out of state; also, many calls from people in town. Torchy,
Chuck, and their son Greg came over in the evening to bring me
a book and card and some special hugs. Bless them all, Lord, for
taking the time to encourage and pray for me."

 The rest of the day I wore myself out, pushing hard to get
the house shipshape, wash all the bedding, etc. When I would
begin to poop out, I would push on, telling myself that I would
have plenty of time to rest. In fact, I knew I would sleep the
entire next day and then sleep and be waited on for several days.
I decided that it was just possible, after the day I had put in, that
the hospital would seem like a luxury hotel.
 In my moments of dread, I would sing, "You Are My Hiding
Place." Concentrating on the verse, "Whenever I am afraid, I
will trust in you," I asked the Lord to assist me in that trust. I
also reminded Him what a megawimp I was (in case it had slipped
His mind) and asked Him to minimize the physical pain and
discomfort for me.
 I finally collapsed into bed, snuggling into Jerry's arms. We
prayed together and I drifted off into a peaceful sleep.

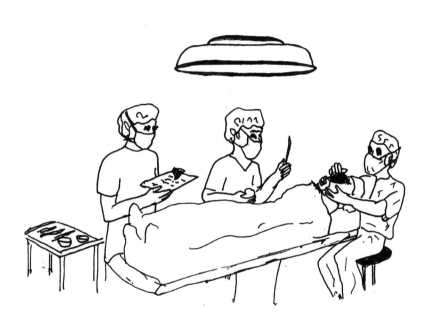

Chapter Thirteen
Under the Knife

The clock radio went off at 4:30 A.M. Jerry had to coax me out of bed—I was in no hurry to start the day! I much preferred my warm, safe bed, with my husband beside me. Finally, I could stall no longer and ventured into the shower. As I dried off, I paused in front of the mirror to study my body, to have one last look at my breast. I didn't even mind the little dent left from the biopsy. It was beautiful to me just the way it was. I felt such sadness looking at the body I was accustomed to—for the last time.

On the day of my surgery, January 9, Spokane had its worst snowstorm of the year. As we drove to the hospital, I wondered if anyone would brave the storm to sit with my men as they spent the long day in the waiting room. Having gone through lengthy surgeries with both Jerry and Michael, I knew how beneficial companionship could be in occupying the anxious mind and passing the time. Michael still had a week left of his Christmas break from college, and David had stayed home from school. The boys wanted to lend their love and support. We needed to be together; we felt stronger as a unit. Most of all, I think they wanted to support their father, to be with him as the difficult hours passed.

The loneliest moments of my life were when the nurse called me away from my family and into a small room to undress. Secluded in that room I prayed: "Lord, I feel so alone. No one, not even Jerry, can *really* go through this with me. It's just you and me. I can't do this without you. Please help me!"

Attired in the hospital gown and slippers and holding the back of the gown closed in my fist, I rushed out to sit with my men. Being near them relieved a bit of my anxiety. My sanctuary didn't last long, however, because the nurse came out and said, "Thought you could get away, huh?" (I was certain she must have followed the thunderous pounding of my heart.)

"I need you to come with me," she said. "Your family can come along too." We obediently followed her into the next room, where she got me settled into a hospital bed. As she started my IV, she told me that these moments leading up to the surgery would be the worst part of my ordeal and assured me that I would be fine.

As I lay there quietly, tears rolled down from the corners of my eyes and into my hair. I felt so sorry for my three men. I could see the pain in their eyes as they stood beside me feeling totally helpless. I wished that I were tougher, that I could act like it was no big deal, for their sakes. This was one time in my life that I couldn't summon the wisecracks and humor to relieve my anxiety, or theirs.

Soon, Ronnie and Peggy arrived. I felt a bit more solace since Ronnie has been like a mother to me for many years. As Ronnie bent over to kiss me, she apologized for being late. Peggy's car got stuck in the snow, and they had to dig themselves out.

My men were relieved. They seemed to know I needed some maternal comfort. David took Ronnie aside, hugged her, and with tears in his eyes said, "Thank you so much for coming. You don't know how much this means to me, to us . . . my mom needed you." Ronnie said she could sense that he felt such a burden, not only for me but also for his dad's pain for me.

They all stood around my bed and Ronnie prayed. She thanked the Lord that He was the Great Physician, the Comforter. She asked Him to guide the surgeon's hands. That the

96

surgery would go perfectly with no complications whatsoever. That I would suffer absolutely no side affects from the anesthetic and no pain after the surgery. And that He would calm the hearts of my family.

They came to take me to pre-op. My family, Ronnie, and Peggy followed. There, I saw Dr. Matsumoto and Dr. Cooper. Dr. Cooper closed the curtains around the two of us, then drew blue lines on my breast, abdomen, and under my bellybutton where he would make his incisions. I couldn't bring myself to look. I nervously teased him about playing "connect the dot" on my body. Both of us were aware that my wise cracks were futile attempts to cover my dread. We briefly made eye contact as he left, and I sensed that in spite of the fact that he loved doing this surgical procedure, he was deeply saddened by what I was going through. I can see where a surgeon would *have* to detach emotionally from a patient, especially someone they liked personally, and force themselves to think "clinically" in order to get the job done.

I got back on the bed and as I signed some papers, a nurse in surgical garb who was standing at the foot of my bed winked at me and said, "I just slipped something in your IV to relax you." Although my family says they all kissed me and I responded, the nurse's comment was the last thing I remember.

By 8:30 A.M. I was in surgery. Dr. Matsumoto had started the mastectomy. Dr. Cooper, with Dr. Olmsted assisting him, began preparing my abdomen to reconstruct my new breast. They removed the muscle, skin, and fat in an almond shape, leaving the vein and artery intact for the blood supply.

By 10:30, Dr. Matsumoto had completed his part of the surgery. Dr. Cooper prepared the vein and artery under my arm.

By noon, Dr. Cooper had severed the blood supply from my abdomen. While looking through a floor-mounted microscope, he reattached the vein and artery from my abdomen to the ones under my arm.

By 3:00 P.M., Dr. Olmsted began repairing my abdomen, stretching the top skin down to meet the bottom skin. He sliced a new opening for my navel, brought my navel through, and stitched it to the top skin. As Dr. Olmsted worked on my abdomen, Dr. Cooper shaped my new breast, using the one Dr. Matsumoto had removed as a pattern. He shaved and tapered the underlying muscle and fat, sculpting and creating a new breast to duplicate the one God had originally designed for me.

By 4:30, the surgery was complete. It had taken eight hours to take me apart and put me back together again.

The next thing I remember was Jerine, a nurse and friend of mine, patting my cheek gently and saying, "Do you recognize me, Sweetie? Do you know who I am?" I managed to nod my head. With less than a whisper, I tried to tell her my lips were dry. David was able to understand my mumblings and interpreted for me. Jerine put Vaseline on my lips. She wasn't my nurse that night but was working on the same floor, and it was comforting to know that she was near.

Everyone sounded like they were far away, but I was aware that Jerry, Michael, and David were kissing me goodbye. Since I was settled into my room, they felt comfortable leaving me to rest. They had endured a tough day, perhaps more than I, and went home for some much needed recuperation.

During the night I slept fairly well, in spite of the routine poking and prodding by the nurses. I had my trusty morphine button in hand and used it, although I don't remember any severe pain. I did have a frightening experience that night, however, when a night nurse came in to get me out of bed to go to the bathroom. She refused to take my word that I wasn't to get out of bed until Dr. Cooper gave his consent. She acted like I was trying to make her job difficult, and she wasn't going to allow it! She angrily told me that if I didn't cooperate and get up with her and go to the bathroom, she would catheterize me. Then she said, "Oh, you're already catheterized. What's going on here?" and stormed out of my room. I hoped she was intending to read my chart!

The next morning when Dr. Cooper made his rounds, I was what my grandfather used to call a "stool pigeon." Yup, I finked on that grumpy, highfalutin' nurse. I heard him in the hall telling the morning shift that I was not to get up until he gave the order! Though he was polite, there wasn't even a hint of maybe in his voice. Within minutes there was a sign above my bed that said, "Patient is to remain in a waist-flexed position until otherwise ordered by Dr. Cooper." Next time someone bullies me— I'm calling Dr. Cooper!

(In the night nurse's defense, this was the first time the Free TRAM Flap surgical procedure had ever been done at the hospital. Many medical people—even physicians—hadn't and haven't yet heard of it. I didn't see her again until the next night when she came into my room and apologized for scaring me. She said she didn't realize that I had also had abdominal surgery and explained that it was routine to get mastectomy patients up right away. Even so, it would have been nice if this nurse, who was taking part in my care, had taken time to read my chart!)

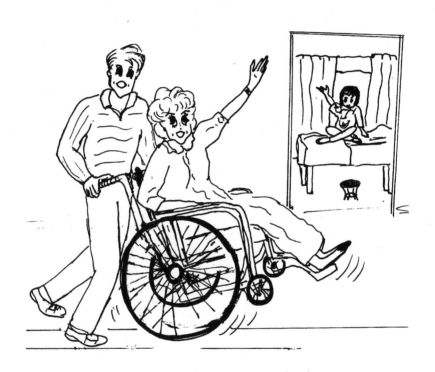

Chapter Fourteen
Hospital Habitation and Hullabaloo

About 7:00 A.M. on the morning following surgery, Jerry came to the hospital on his way to work, and Michael came along with him to spend the day with me. Dr. Cooper had not yet made his rounds, so I told Jerry and Michael about the nurse who demanded a reveille in the middle of the night. I was weak and was fearful that she, or someone else, would try again to drag me out of bed, causing me harm. Jerry stepped outside my room and talked to a nurse about my frightening ordeal. Michael vowed to stay by my side all day long as insurance. Our good-byes said, Jerry left for work, leaving Michael as my guardian angel.

I told Michael that his Christmas break was coming to a rapid close, and I hated to see him spend his remaining time at the hospital. He said, "Mom, you are always there for me. I want to be here for you. I am exactly where I want to be."

Michael was very protective. I drifted in and out, but the sudden ring of the telephone startled me. Since the phone didn't have a volume control, he took it from the nightstand and put it as far away from the bed as the cord would allow, covered it with a pillow, and answered it on the first ring. He was there until evening to provide me with sips of water and encouraging words. He wouldn't even leave me to have lunch, until my friend Marcia arrived and promised to stay by my side until he returned.

Donna arrived about 7:30 A.M., having already taken her husband, Chuck, to the airport for an early flight. When Dr. Matsumoto made his rounds, he was surprised to see Donna and Michael there so early. They waited out in the hall so that Dr. Matsumoto could examine me privately. Because he left the operating room long before Dr. Cooper had finished reconstructing my new breast, he hadn't yet seen the results. In my fog, I hadn't given my new breast much thought. As far as I was aware, Dr. Matsumoto was getting the first peek. He seemed impressed. I took that as a good sign.

Donna filled me in on my lost day. It seems that in spite of the terrible storm, our friends really came through. Joannie, a former head nurse on the orthopedic unit who knew the hospital well, arrived to lend her support and was able to make periodic calls to the operating room for progress reports. Friends from the choir who were on staff at the hospital spent their breaks in the waiting room. The room was filled all day with various friends coming and going. Ron and Connie even brought *cookies!* I accused them of having a stinking party while I was under the knife! No fair! I really hate it when I miss out on fun. The party was in my honor (sort of), and I didn't even get a crummy cookie!

Dr. Cooper came into the waiting room with a big smile on his face and told my family and friends that my surgery couldn't have gone better. All had gone perfectly, with no complications. Donna tells me that Jerry and Pastor Rich shed some heartfelt tears of relief together. I believe that my breast cancer experience brought back some painful buried emotions for Rich. As a young fourteen-year-old boy, he had watched helplessly as breast cancer, in its cruelty, robbed him of his mother.

Lynn came in later that morning with a stuffed cow, one that mooed when turned upside down. Lynnie loves cows and has a massive collection. I felt honored, first of all, that she would endow me with a cow; and secondly, that it actually remained in my custody when she left the hospital cowless, proving again, that we were, and are, "udderly" pals!

At one point, Lynn, Donna, and I were having a tête-à-tête in which I boasted of how alert and clever I was, not drifting off as is customary for a patient the day following a long surgery. They looked at each other and burst into hysterical laughter, apparently I wasn't quite as perky as I thought! They accused me of stopping in mid-sentence to take a five-minute nap, then waking up to finish my sentence while they were already onto the next subject. I told them it wasn't nice to make fun of a sick person! Their job was to spoil and pamper me! Besides, I'm not sure their version of that day is all that reliable. I had quite a few guests, and I'm sure I was a most gracious hostess!

Among my visitors that afternoon were Julie and her daughter, Lindsey. They brought with them a grocery bag filled with snacks for Jerry and the boys to consume during their visits. What a great gift idea for someone in the hospital who has visiting sons with enormous appetites! When Julie called the day before my surgery, I was having a difficult moment, and she read me Psalm 91:14-16. I wrote it on an index card inserting my name:

> "Because Sherry loves me," says the Lord, "I will rescue her; I will protect her, for she acknowledges my name. Sherry will call upon me, and I will answer her; I will be with her in trouble, I will deliver her and honor her. With long life will I satisfy her and show her my salvation."

I kept this index card with me until someone took it out of my hand after I was anesthetized. Though I never expected to see it again, I found it in my belongings when I returned home.

Julie, a good friend of ours, works as a counselor, and is a colleague of my counselor, Rachel. Rachel had been helping me deal with the trauma that accompanies cancer and the assault on womanhood that a mastectomy brings. She was delighted and excited when I discovered the Free TRAM Flap. When moments of fear would squeeze my heart and I would have doubts about the reconstruction I had chosen, she would gently remind me that it seemed like the Lord had taken me by the hand and led me to Dr. Cooper and this innovative procedure. In fear, I couldn't run away—at least not without giving it serious thought and prayer.

Rachel was scheduled to be in Hawaii with her husband at the time of my surgery but promised to pray for me in earnest. She called Julie at the office to check on my progress and asked Julie to inform me that she would be calling me at the hospital at a designated time. I have always loved and appreciated Rachel for her Godly counsel. I was especially touched by her thoughtful and encouraging call from Hawaii.

Rachel's call was one of many kindnesses extended to me during my cancer ordeal. It seems that when we are really burdened with the struggles of life, the Lord manages to send us encouragement in some unforeseen way. These unexpected blessings were a delight to me, and they are dear memories.

In spite of my scare that first night, the hospital care that I received was very good. Rhonda is the nurse I remember the most. She fed me broth and encouraged me with kindness and a good sense of humor.

One of the things I hated the most was that contraption I had to draw a breath through several times a day. I could never get that stupid ball up as high as they wanted. If they had provided more incentive and had told me what the prize was for sucking the ball clear to the top, I might have been better at it! With *my* luck, winning the prize would have meant a free enema, or worse, getting more blood drawn! I wonder if they had any "Blue Ribbon Champion Contraption Suckers" on my floor.

Another thing bugged me. I would be entertaining guests, basking in the glory of being pampered and spoiled, when a nurse would think it was a great opportunity to show off my coughing ability—a grand way to entertain! Since Dr. Cooper had just dug around in my tummy and found a whole boob to take out and stick on my chest, coughing wasn't my idea of a good time! It did help, however, when nurse Rhonda instructed me to press a pillow to my abdomen. (My nurses seemed to have a real thing about coughing and sucking! I bet parties at their houses are a real blast!)

A smiling Dr. Matsumoto came into my room during his rounds one morning. "Good news!" he said. "Your lymph nodes are clear. You don't have to have chemotherapy." A definite answer to prayer; things were starting to look up!

Donna spent many hours at the hospital caring for me. Reflecting on those days, she believes that she *needed* to be there for me. As a fourteen-year-old girl, she witnessed her mother's slow and painful demise from breast cancer. Her life then was spinning out of control. She didn't know what to do or how to handle her fears and emotions. As she loved, nurtured, and served me, she was able to work through many of her unresolved issues and emotions. (It has always seemed odd to me that both Rich and Donna, two of my dearest friends, lost their mothers at the same tender age of fourteen, and to the same dreaded disease.)

An oven-roasted chicken breast with a baked potato for lunch on Saturday was my first solid food, and I scarfed it down in record time. Nothing ever tasted so good! My tummy was full and I was regaining my strength. I sat up in a chair, and Donna brushed my hair while the nurse changed my sheets. Once she had made me "borderline presentable," she took me on my first stroll. I walked a bit bent over, and with a mustache and a cigar I would have been a dead ringer for Groucho Marx!

That Saturday afternoon I was thrilled when Jerry's dad and his friend Sophie popped in to surprise us after driving two hours from Lewiston, Idaho. They spent some time with me, then took Jerry and the boys to dinner. Before leaving for home the next day, they returned to the hospital to stay with me while Jerry and the boys attended church.

Sunday morning I had my first shower, shampoo, and yes, I shaved my legs. After breakfast, I was sitting up in a chair having some coffee when Dr. Cooper made his rounds. I told him how popular my new breast was, that after viewing it everyone would gasp and say, "It's beautiful. It's geometrically perfect. It's amazing!"

He teasingly said, "Maybe you ought to charge a buck a peek?" Why hadn't *I* thought of that?

Dr. Cooper felt I was doing well enough to go home the next day, Monday—and I was ready. I missed being home and knew it would be easier, especially for Jerry. Actually, I have always suspected that the nurses paid him big bucks to discharge me. Once I was feeling semi-perky, I didn't care to stay in bed anymore. It just isn't *fun* to be in a little room, alone and bored. So, naturally, it made perfect sense to me to join the evening nurses at the nurses' station! I have always wondered if they were tempted to drug me and tie me to the bed!

As I have said before, mine was the first Free TRAM Flap done in Spokane, and word traveled fast of this wonderful innovative reconstruction. My new body part was the subject of so much curiosity that I soon developed a strange clinical detachment. I had to. It got to the point that when someone in a white uniform came into my room, I got ready for "show and tell." Wouldn't you know, toward the end of my stay a lady in white walked in. I was getting ready for "show and tell" when I realized that instead of a stethoscope, she had a mop! I decided that Housekeeping probably wasn't all that interested—although she might have been.

Sunday evening Jerry and Michael had to do some last minute shopping before Michael flew back to college the next day. They made the mistake of leaving David and me (two sanguines) unsupervised. I talked David into swiping a wheelchair and taking me on a joy ride. We had a great time until we got back to my room, where Jerry and Michael (the more sensible of the four of us) were waiting. They were looking very stern. David said, "Uh oh, we're busted!" We tried to convince them of the deep shame we felt in our hearts for our transgression, but for some strange reason, I don't think they bought it.

As I recall, this was not the first time David and I have found "trouble" together. Just before Michael went away to college for the first time, the boys and I had been shopping for some last minute things before the trip. At the check stand of a local store, Michael mentioned other things we had to do before he left. The cashier asked where he was going, and before he could tell her that he was going away to college, I said sadly, "He's going to prison." Before Michael had a chance to respond in protest, his brother said, "Yes, it's a family disgrace. He was caught running naked in the mall!" When we got in the car to leave, David and I got a lecture. I don't remember what was said exactly, probably something like, "You don't ever say the word *naked* in public!"

More times than not, the joke is on me! When David was in Middle School he told the kids that his mother was a 300-pound biker who wore leather and rode with the Hell's Angels motorcycle club. He added that he was my pride and joy, and they'd better treat him with respect because I had a temper! Then he came home and told *me* that the kids couldn't wait to meet me. *How sweet,* I thought. When I arrived at school for Parent Hot Lunch Day, there was quite a reception committee in the hall. I think they were disappointed. I would have dressed the part had he informed me! Of course, I probably would have had to get tough with a Hell's Angel in order to "borrow" the outfit. (Sigh.) What a mother won't do for the love of her child!

Jerry especially appreciates sanguine behavior when we go for a family outing and, while stopped at a red light, David gets an uncontrollable urge to roll down the window and bark and howl like a dog, or when he gets out of the car to stretch and greet people in the other cars.

Honestly, he *really* doesn't belong in an institution. He's just a teenage sanguine. It's a condition of his temperament that possibly is accelerated during puberty!

Our adventure over, my three men tucked me into bed. I had a headache after the wheelchair ride (must have been too exciting). The door was slightly ajar, and the only light in the room came from the hall. Jerry was sitting on my left, holding my hand; Michael was holding my right hand; and David was standing at the head of my bed, gently stroking my face. No one spoke. I felt such love poured out on me by those three who own my heart. They are the family that God gave me; I was so grateful for the *gift* of their love and the joy they each bring to my heart. I told them how much I loved them and how wonderful it was to have them all there loving me. David said, "Yes, Mom, this is one of those 'Kodak moments.'" We all started to laugh, which I don't recommend while lying on your back after just having had abdominal surgery. Leave it to David to spice up a precious and tender family moment!

The next morning, Dr. Cooper removed the two drains that were in my breast but left two in my abdomen as souvenirs. He said I was doing great and signed my discharge papers.

I had a male nurse that morning who kindly offered to help me with a shower. I know it was just part of his job, but I wasn't quite ready for that yet and politely declined. I told him that I would wait until I got home—I needed my rubber ducky.

Jerry arrived to spring me from "da joint." My wheelchair ride to the lobby sure wasn't the daring spree I'd had the night before. The nurse's driving didn't compare to David's. She didn't even pop one wheelie!

Finally! I was in the car and on my way home with Jerry! *Home sweet home,* I thought, *here I come!*

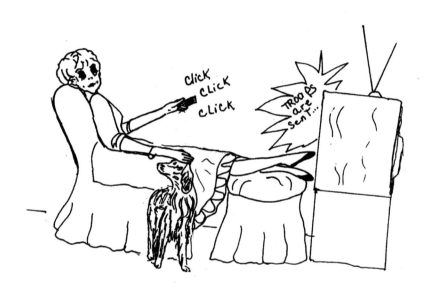

Chapter Fifteen

There's No Place Like Home . . . and Desert Storm

After a snowy ride home, Jerry tucked me into bed, brought my things in from the car, and loaded it back up with Michael's belongings. Michael and I only had a few moments together before Jerry drove him to the airport for his return to college. As Michael lay on the bed next to me, he held my hand and expressed his reluctance to leave. I assured him that even though I looked a little wimpy, a few days at home and I would be ice skating, playing the flute, and jogging to the mall and back.

He said, "Mom, you have never done any of those things in your life!"

"Oh yeah, I forgot!" I replied. "I *could* take them up, you know. Stranger things have happened!"

"I don't think so, Mom, not that strange." He kissed me goodbye and took off for sunny California.

Jerry didn't want me to be alone, so he called Ron and Connie to come over and "booby-sit" me. They arrived just minutes after Jerry and Michael left for the airport. I asked for references, but it was their first "booby-sitting" job, and they didn't have a reference portfolio compiled as yet. I wasn't too sure about their qualifications but decided to let them stay anyway. Besides, what could I do? Jerry had ordered me to stay in bed and had left the door unlocked. (Luckily, there were no axe murdering fiends lurking in the neighborhood.) They brought in a couple of chairs from the kitchen and sat by my bed. I teased them about bringing cookies to the hospital waiting room for my "surgery party," and I, the reason for the party, went cookieless!

We have enjoyed a wonderful friendship with Ron and Connie that dates back to when our children were little. Connie and I spent some white-knuckled moments together watching her son Travis and my David do outrageous stunts on skateboard ramps. We wanted them to wear crash dummy outfits, or at least to tie pillows around their bodies and limbs, but they wouldn't go for it. I guess it spoils the fun if the kamikaze aspect is eliminated. To their credit (or skill) neither one of them suffered any injuries worse than a bad scrape. They probably worked their guardian angels into a frenzy. I pictured frazzled angels, with their halos drooping down over one eye, darting around with their arms extended, trying to prevent the boys from killing themselves. I just know they begged God for an easier duty, like a motorcycle daredevil or a bomb repair man.

Michael, and Ron and Connie's daughter, Tina have been lifelong pals too, although they didn't partake in daredevil, death-defying, hobbies—as far as we knew, anyway.

When Ron and Connie took their leave, I shifted my position to get more comfortable. A few minutes later my back felt wet, and I realized that I had rolled onto the bulb of one of the drains left in my abdomen. The lid had popped off, and it had leaked all over the bed. I burst into tears and told Jerry what I had done. I was emotionally and physically exhausted, and this tipped me over the edge. Jerry did his best to console me and quickly helped me out of my wet clothes and onto a chair. He stripped the bed, threw the bedding into the wash, helped me with a shower, settled me on the couch, and ran to the pharmacy to get my pain and sleeping medication. My poor husband was spent. He had to juggle work, the boy's needs, and my needs—all the while neglecting his own. Jerry had been struggling with his own fears about his lifelong partner's cancer, and although he would never admit it, I imagine that he was grieving the loss of my breast from a husband's perspective. He also had concerns not only for my physical health but for my emotional health as well. It was a heavy load for him to carry, and I could see in his eyes that he was beyond exhaustion.

He finally sat down with me in the living room at about 11:00 that night. My heart was broken for him and I said, "Honey, you are so exhausted. I'm sorry to be putting you through all of this." His eyes filled with tears as he snapped at me, "Don't you dare say that to me! I am so grateful that you are alive and home with me. I'm thrilled to have the *chance* to take care of you!"

With Michael back in college and David in bed, we were finally alone. Though worn and spent in many ways, it was wonderful to be together in our home. A simple thing taken for granted for so many years felt like a treasured gift: to be able to just hold each other again, and rest. It's true. The simple things in life *are* the most precious. Unfortunately, sometimes it takes a trial for us to realize that.

As we went to bed, Jerry tried to make me comfortable with pillows while he gave my night orders. I was not to try to get up to go to the bathroom or do anything else without his help. I was to wake him for any need. His order was unnecessary, however, because every time I moved a muscle, he awoke. In spite of everything, the night went pretty well. The medication helped me to sleep, and the pillows helped to prop me on my side, yet sort of on my tummy—my favorite position.

The next morning, Jerry fixed breakfast, got David off to school, and emptied my drains, as he would do twice daily. I was so thankful for his medical training in the Navy, and later as an operating room technician. He isn't a bit squeamish and has always been so quick to care for me or the boys when needed. I, however, am a wimp and tend to get weak in the knees at the sight of a hangnail. Our boys were kind enough to save their biggest boyhood boo-boos for when their dad was around. I have always considered that very thoughtful of them. Or, was it that they somehow knew that a mother who would faint into a state of unconscious oblivion wouldn't be very helpful?

Jerry had arranged a schedule of friends to "booby-sit" so I wouldn't be alone. I would have been fine alone, but he insisted that I have someone with me, so I decided to think of it as a miniparty every day. I did need help getting off the couch, until I learned the right *roll-off* maneuvers. A section of my stomach muscle had become a part of my new breast, and the muscle that remained was weak for quite a while.

I settled on the couch with the remote control in my hand. My men let me hold it when they're not home. Male-type people can get quite territorial when it comes to the remote control. I think the key word here is *control*. (The television remote control is an interesting device. Lynn says that you can tell when a boy becomes a man, and it has nothing to do with an increase in testosterone—it's when he starts clutching the remote control to his chest. It's one of those "guy things." Lynn talks about her father-in-law falling asleep in the recliner with the remote control firmly gripped to his chest. Her mother-in-law managed to slip it out of his clutches and hide it. He woke up in a panic and went on a desperate search. He was just about to call one of those TV shows, *Missing Remotes,* or *America's Most Wanted Devices,* when she decided to put it where he could find it. She did. He did. Immense relief flooded over him.)

Since Lynn, my "booby-sitter" for the day, had not yet arrived, I mustered up some testosterone and flipped on the television to find that during the night President Bush had declared war on Saddam Hussein. I had been out of touch for nearly a week. I hadn't watched television, listened to a radio, or even read a paper while at the hospital. Visitors usually don't bring up an impending war when they visit a hospital patient—that would be tacky. It was quite a shock to realize that we were at war. I watched, feeling heartbroken and fearful for what could happen.

Lynn arrived. I snapped out of it and turned off the television. Nothing like a sanguine! Lynn's presence is very commanding. She can even make a war go away. Maybe President Bush should have hired her!

Lynn brought lunch, did the laundry, put a roast dinner in the oven, played hostess to the visitors, and made us all laugh. Lynnie's creed is that laughter and chocolate are remedies that can cure just about anything. When you think of it, it's not a bad creed.

Every day that week was similar: friends, food, and frivolity. Generous friends and neighbors brought in meals. Ronnie scrubbed my floor, serenading me with song as she worked. I found it very strange, and difficult, to sit by and allow someone else to perform my household duties. However, I was grateful for each thing that our friends did because it took some of the pressure off of Jerry. I had joked with Dr. Cooper, dramatically slipping the back of my hand up to my forehead, and asked him to order no housework for a year. I claimed that housework would put unnecessary strain on my new boob. I asked him to write a prescription for chocolate and old movies. He played along, but I never left his office with that prescription. The truth was that I was longing to get back to normal. I wanted to take care of my home and family so Jerry would have the option of clutching that remote to his chest after a hard day at work and be able to rest.

There was nothing on television but war. Desert Storm. I was working on regaining my strength, and I needed to keep a positive attitude. The war was making that a challenge. I didn't seem to have concentration enough to read, possibly the result of the anesthetic given to me during surgery. So, Jerry went to

115

the library and checked out a bunch of old black and white movies. When I had no visitors, I spent the day with Cary Grant, David Niven, or other hunks from the forties. It was not only a wonderful way to pass the time, but a great escape.

I had looked *down* at my new breast and displayed it to the "oohs" and "ahhs" of curious "girl-type" friends and, of course, the hospital staff; but I had been avoiding a close self-examination. I finally mustered up the courage to look straight on at myself in the mirror. I unbuttoned my robe in front of the bathroom mirror, with Jerry by my side. He smiled and said, "See, it's beautiful, isn't it?"

It really was! Geometrically it matched the other side perfectly. Just as Dr. Cooper had forewarned, however, it was tight and it would be for a short while. I joked that it looked like I had a forty-four-year-old boob and a fourteen-year-old boob. But I knew that it would continue to relax and get softer, and within six months I would once again have a matched set! My eyes welled up with tears from a grateful heart. God had truly answered my prayer to be whole after my surgery. Jerry put his arms around me, and as he held me he said, "I think your new breast looks wonderful. Dr. Cooper is an artist!" I certainly agreed.

A week after my release from the hospital, my good friend Judy took me to see Dr. Cooper, and best of all, get those annoying drains taken out. It was good to see Dr. Cooper again. He was pleased with the outcome of my surgery. He pulled out the drains and removed some stitches from my abdomen. I was sitting on the examination table, and he asked if I had any problems or questions.

I said, "I love my new breast, but I do have this one kinda problem."

He looked concerned and said, "What is it?"

"Well," I said, "every time I get hungry, my boob growls!"

He laughed and said, "I don't recall putting any stomach parts up there."

"Are you sure?" I whined. "I just know I'm going to be humiliated with embarrassment at church, or somewhere where boob growling would be highly inappropriate."

He grinned at me, "I'm sure."

Because Dr. Cooper was still in the Air Force Reserves, I told him I was concerned about Desert Storm and hoped he wouldn't be called into active duty. He and his family were hoping the same thing. (He did get called up and spent about four weeks at Travis Air Force Base in California; but, he never had to leave the states.)

I gave him a hug goodbye and thanked him again for the beautiful job he did on my reconstruction. Although I was becoming a bit more vertical, I still resembled Groucho Marx's bent over gait and must have been a sight as I made my next appointment and exited his office.

Being rather pooped, I couldn't wait to get home and wondered if I would ever get my strength back.

I was increasingly able to do more around the house and had graduated from my robe into sweats. The excitement was wearing off. I was alone more and began to get depressed.

Although cancer had certainly been a monumental concern before my surgery, a large part of my anxiety was over the trauma of the mastectomy. That was over now, and thanks to Dr. Cooper's skill, I felt like my body was still intact. I had a few scars that would fade in time, but the emotional wound inside me that accompanies cancer was beginning to fester.

One morning I was alone in the house, sitting in the bathtub, looking at my scars. I was feeling relieved that the surgery was behind me, realizing all I had been through, and having a good cry. Tears can be very cleansing, so the bathtub seemed the appropriate place to let my tears cleanse my soul. The telephone rang. I picked up the cordless phone that I had placed on the floor next to the tub. It was a *friend* who said she could tell by my voice that I wasn't the "cheerful Sherry" she was accustomed to and asked what was wrong. I told her that I was having a delayed reaction to the trauma of cancer. She more or less told me to buck up, scolded me, and said that the pain of her divorce was much worse than cancer or losing a breast. I was stunned and hurt that she would hurl such a "shame on you" attitude at me. Before ending the conversation, I did manage to tell her that even if the two situations could be compared, I didn't think she was qualified to make that judgment, since she had not experienced breast cancer.

In comparing notes with other breast cancer survivors, I have found it bewildering and appaling what women will say to one another. "At least you're not married!" "Be grateful you don't have any children." "Be thankful you're small busted; it won't be as traumatic as it would for someone like me with bigger breasts." "At least you're still alive." "Even if your hair does fall out, it always grows back." "If it were me, I would just want to die. I would no longer feel like a woman. I would refuse the surgery."

There is a bit of truth to *some* of these statements; however, when you are facing breast cancer, *you need encouragement.* It doesn't help to have someone minimize the significance of your anguish.

Of course, there are always the ones who love to tell horror stories of people who suffered great pain and agony before their death. It really isn't helpful to hear about your sister's husband's brother's wife's cousin twice removed who vomited uncontrollably day and night after chemotherapy. Who not only lost her hair but all of her eyelashes and her eyebrows. And her husband deserted her after her mastectomy. Then her dog got hit by a Hostess Twinkie truck, went into convulsions, and died. We would rather hear success stories; be taken to lunch; be given a hug (we are not contagious); receive a humorous book or an entertaining video; or receive an offer for a ride to the doctor or a chemotherapy treatment. And yet, if we need to cry, just lend a sympathetic ear and offer a prayer. Never, "Buck up, you haven't suffered anything like I have." Or, "Let me tell you about my poor Aunt Hilda who barfed so much her entire spleen jumped right out of her mouth!"

Before my surgery, another *friend* said to me, "I wouldn't go through that reconstruction. I'm not as concerned with *my* body image as you are." Well, shame on me!

I was struck speechless at the time, but now my response would be: "We are all different, and the women who choose reconstruction are not consumed with vanity or lacking in spiritual depth. They are just different. I truly hope you never find out, but I'm not sure you can be confident of how you would react if you were told that you had cancer and to save your life your breast must be amputated."

We are women who need to encourage and support one another, especially when we have an enemy like breast cancer attacking at an alarming rate. We can't be judging each other's reactions and choices. There is no right or wrong decision when it comes to reconstruction. Whether reconstruction is chosen or not, each option is equally acceptable. It's a very personal choice.

Most everyone in my life was totally supportive and thrilled to know that this innovative procedure was available, and they said that they would choose it for themselves in a heartbeat. It was wonderful and reassuring to hear *those* needed words of encouragement. Breast cancer is quite enough to deal with on its own. Those unfortunate enough to be going through that valley certainly don't need judgment and horror stories.

Lynn took me to my first follow-up appointment with Dr. Matsumoto. I was absolutely stir crazy from being housebound for what seemed like an eternity. I was so excited and felt like a prisoner "gettin' sprung from da' joint." When Judy took me to see Dr. Cooper, I was still in the "patient who just had surgery mode." Then I felt wimpy and weak. But this time I was feeling stronger and ready to experience life again.

I put on makeup and fussed over my hair. I wasn't yet allowed to wear a bra, so I wore a blue satiny night shirt that could easily pass for a day shirt. I slipped into my black stirrup pants and put on some jewelry. I was, quite simply, darling! I had been looking very undarling lately, so darling was a fun change.

Seeing Lynn's car pull up in the driveway was so exciting, I would have jumped up and down—if I could have. I put on my coat and we headed out the back door. As we were getting in the car, Gaylen, my neighbor, was out in his driveway across the street.

He said, "Sherry, it's good to see you. You look great!"

I replied, "Thanks, it's my first time out of the house!"

He hollered at Lynn, "You be careful with her!"

I got in the car, buckled up, and grinned at Lynn. She burst out laughing, "I can tell already, this is going to be quite an experience!"

"I certainly hope so!" I replied.

We took off down the street with me beaming from ear to ear, waiting to experience life on the outside. A chipmunk ran across the road and went scurrying up a tree. I screamed, "Lynn, look, a chipmunk! Isn't he cute?"

After she got her heart going again, she said, "Yes, it's so clever how they can just run across a road like that."

"He's probably going to get his stash of nuts," I said. "There will be a chipmunk party in the neighborhood tonight!"

We headed down the street where a crew was doing some roadwork. I was happy to see these nice men fixing the road, so I smiled and waved at them, and they smiled and waved back.

"See, Lynnie," I grinned. "Everyone is glad I'm out of the house."

"I can tell you right now," Lynn said, "I'm experiencing great bliss, equal to none other in my life!" As we sat at a stoplight, a Roto Rooter truck crossed in front of us.

I said, "You know, Lynnie, I have never appreciated Roto Rooter trucks until this very moment."

She said, "I don't know why. I myself have always found them quite appealing." (Conversations between sanguines don't necessarily have to make sense).

We arrived at the medical building, and a nice older gentleman held the door open for us. "Thank you, sir," I beamed. "This is my first day out of the house since my surgery."

"Oh," he said, wondering, I suspect, if my "surgery" had been a lobotomy.

As we all got on the elevator, a lady kindly asked what floor we needed.

"Six, please," I replied. Lynn grinned and jabbed me with her elbow. The confused lady looked at the buttons and then laughed because there were only three floors.

We got off the elevator and went into Dr. Matsumoto's office. As I waited for him, I recalled the heaviness that was in my heart the first time I visited his office and realized how much lighter my heart felt this time. I was very grateful to have the surgery behind me.

He came in, examined my breast and abdomen, and said everything looked good. He wanted to know if I had any questions.

I, of course, said, "Well, Dr. Matsumoto, I do have this one kinda problem."

He put on his concerned doctor face and said, "Yes, what is it?"

I said, "Well, whenever I get h. . . did you know that your tie is crooked?"

"No," he said, straightening it. "What was it you were saying?"

"Well," I said, "It's really kind of embarrassing. It's my new breast. You see, every time I get really h. . . you know, that tie still isn't straight."

"I just got out of surgery," he said apologetically, looking in the mirror this time to straighten his tie. "What is it that's bothering you?"

"I'm sorry. It's really very difficult to talk about," I said sadly.

"Its okay, just take your time," he reassured me.

"Well, it's just that since the TRAM Flap was taken from my abdomen, now, when I get hungry, my boob growls!"

He rolled his eyes as he laughed and smacked me on the knee!

As we left his office, he told me to come back in a year—or did he say, "Don't you dare come back in here for a year!" I can't remember exactly.

We were on our way down the hall when I decided that we should stop and see Deloras, a friend who worked for a doctor in the building. She had previously told me that Dr. Slick had seen a botched TRAM Flap that had been done several years earlier. When she talked to him about my choosing that form of reconstruction, he had expressed concern.

We walked into the doctor's office and noticed that the nice gentleman who had opened the door for us when we arrived at the building was sitting in the waiting room, reading a newspaper. When he looked up and saw us, he raised the paper over his face. He probably just wanted to be careful not to miss anything on the bottom of the page, but maybe he was hiding.

Deloras was tickled to see us and went back to ask the doctor if he wanted to see how well the surgery turned out. She returned and said the doctor and his nurse were both anxious to see the outcome. They were amazed and relieved to see how well and healthy it looked. He thanked me for being willing to show him and wanted to know the name of the plastic surgeon.

As we drove out of the parking lot, Lynn asked if I felt up to lunch at Percy's. I said yes, it seemed like forever since we'd had a lunch date.

I took off my coat and started sipping my herbal tea when Lynn started laughing.

"I can't believe we're sitting here at Percy's with you in your nightie, and braless to boot!"

I replied rather smugly, "I don't usually wear a bra when I'm in my nightie, regardless of where I am at the time. Of course, this *is* my first visit to a restaurant in my nightie, but it *is* kind of comfortable. I just might make it a habit!"

We had a wonderful, carefree lunch, just like in the B.C. days (before cancer). No one even suspected that my attire was not quite appropriate for the occasion.

After lunch, we went to the Bible bookstore across the mall from Percy's. We were browsing around when Lynn looked at me and said, "You're sinking fast. I'd better get you home."

She was right. I was starting to wind down at a rapid pace—too much zaniness for one day, at least in my condition.

I don't ever remember being so happy to be out with a friend. I felt free, giddy, like a ton of weight had been lifted from my shoulders. I guess that accounted for the extra frivolity of the day.

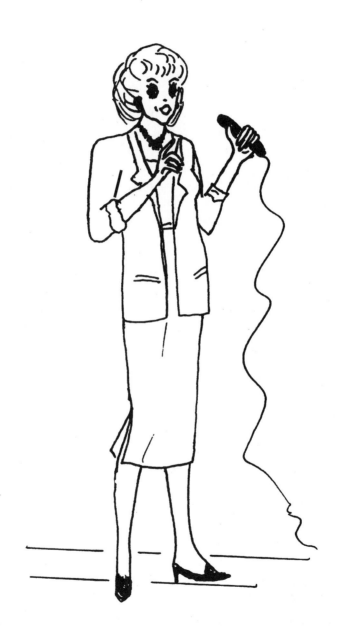

Chapter Sixteen

Spreading the Good News!

I was healing and feeling more like me every day. Being able to go to David's basketball games once again did wonders for my spirits. I still tired easily, though, and had to pace myself.

I met Delora the year I graduated from Bible Study Fellowship. She was in the process of going to college to become a counselor. I was impressed that she was doing both B.S.F. and counseling classes at the same time. Delora heard about my ordeal and called to invite me to lunch at Percy's. On our lunch date she told me her schooling was completed and that she had specialized in counseling cancer survivors. She started a support group and invited me to join them.

I told her that I was still struggling at times but thought I could handle it with the help of Jerry and my friends. If I felt I needed to talk to a counselor, I could talk to Rachel or Julie, two very special counselor friends who are always there for me. As Delora and I talked, she said that it was terrific I had such wonderful support, but as much as my family and friends loved me, they didn't really understand what I was going through. She explained that sometimes it helps to talk to women who are walking the same walk. Sometimes we hold back feelings and fears because we don't want to burden or worry our loved ones. She also urged me to attend the support group so I could tell the women about my reconstruction. She felt it would be an encouragement to the group to know there was an alternative to implants.

I decided to take her up on her offer. It wouldn't hurt to try it a couple of times, and I wanted to inform as many women as possible about the Free TRAM Flap. I knew I had good news that I couldn't possibly keep to myself. To do so would be selfish and unfair.

I attended the group a few times, meeting a variety of women each week: an attorney, a teacher, an artist, single women, mothers, and grandmothers. Most of them had breast cancer. A few were dealing with other forms of cancer. There was laughter. For example, they claimed that one of the advantages of chemotherapy was the amount of money saved on shampoo. I confessed my fear of shaving under my arm, which was numb. I was afraid I would cut myself and bleed to death. I could just see the headlines: *Suicide Attempt, Woman Slashes Pit!* They assured me that this was a common fear, and one lady divulged that she didn't shave for about nine months. Boy, she must have had quite a crop!

There were also tears of frustration and anxiety. As we talked about our hopes, our fears, and our struggles, I sensed a very real camaraderie.

On my second visit to the support group, Delora asked me to share about my reconstruction. The group listened with amazement and curiosity. When I showed them my reconstruction, one of the women burst into tears.

She was furious, "Why wasn't I told about this?" She said, "My mastectomy was just two weeks ago. I would have had this surgery if someone had only told me! With the implant controversy, my doctor advised me against having any reconstruction, saying that in five years I wouldn't even miss my breast!"

We were all stunned and irate when we heard this doctor's ignorant, thoughtless statement!

Won't miss it in five years? How dare he say something like that! I wondered aloud how he would feel if a part of *his* anatomy, a part of his masculinity, had been chopped off. Would it be missed in five years!? I tried to console her by assuring her that it wasn't too late. She could still have the reconstruction. It can be done several years after the mastectomy. She replied that it would mean more time off work, and she couldn't deal with putting herself through another surgery at that point.

I didn't see this lady again and don't know if she ever had reconstruction, but I will never forget her. Her anguish broke my heart, affecting me in two distinct ways. First, I was so totally grateful that I had found Dr. Cooper and the Free TRAM Flap *and* that I had found out in time to have it incorporated into the same procedure as the mastectomy, eliminating a second surgery. Thankfully, I didn't have to experience her anguish, her exasperation. Second, I left with a fierce determination to do whatever I could to inform women of this option.

It's most likely that her doctor didn't deliberately withhold this information from her; he may not have known. It's also possible that he had heard of it but didn't know there was a plastic surgeon in Spokane who had this specialized training.

I was suddenly on a crusade. I was compelled to spread the news to doctors, to let them know there was wonderful information for them to tell their heartbroken breast cancer patients. They could explain to them that the implant controversy didn't mean there was no hope for replacing their absent breast. There was not only hope. They had a much better option!

How would I accomplish this? Would I have to visit every doctor in town personally?

"Hi, my name is Sherry. Ya wanna see my terrific new boob?" I think not! They might call someone to come and take me away. I had to find another approach.

127

At the same time, I knew women had to be informed. In my zeal, I wanted to shout at them from the rooftops or accost them in the grocery store. Well, maybe I wouldn't go quite that far. After all, some of my credibility might suffer if I exclaimed this wonderful news attired in a straitjacket!

I did visit a few doctors I knew, and they were quite impressed with the results of my reconstructive surgery. They commented that it was very natural looking, geometrically matched my other breast, and that it was especially good that it was my own tissue. They asked who had done my surgery, and I was more than happy to tell them, leaving with them Dr. Cooper's card.

One doctor I visited said that, as a man, he couldn't understand why a woman would opt for two scars instead of just one. Well, personally, I really don't care about the scar on my abdomen. What's important to me is that I have a breast! The scar on my lower abdomen couldn't be more insignificant to me.

As I said before, when talking about my breast and showing it to doctors, I was strangely detached—it all seemed very clinical. Even so, I felt uncomfortable visiting the few doctors' offices that I did, so I started telephoning hospitals. I was able to set up some speaking engagements for Dr. Cooper. He asked me to put something together from the patient's perspective and join him in the presentations.

The first thing we did was a "Continuing Medical Education Seminar" for doctors at a local hospital. I was quite nervous about that one. I had been a public speaker for several years, but only to women—a group of doctors was another story.

I have heard it said that speakers who feel nervous speaking in front of a group should picture the audience naked. A lady, such as I, couldn't possibly do something so crass; it wouldn't be proper. So, I decided that if fear got the best of me, I would picture the male members of the audience sitting there in loud, colorful boxer shorts. I figured guys never look *too* scary in boxer shorts.

The hospital provided lunch, and Dr. Cooper spoke first, using a slide presentation. He gave information about implants and a history of the evolution of the Free TRAM Flap. It seems that women, mastectomy patients, came up with the idea. At the very inception of the mastectomy as a surgery, women began asking their doctors, "Why don't you just take this fat from my stomach, or thighs, or bottom, and reconstruct a new breast?"

Most women seem to produce a little extra as they age, and it made sense to them. You not only acquire a new breast, you also get rid of some unwanted fat! Great concept, don't you think? Plastic surgeons began trying it in the late seventies and have been perfecting it for years. Then why hasn't the general public heard of it? Good question!

Some of Dr. Cooper's slides were of the actual surgery and were very graphic. I had to look away. Before my surgery, Dr. Cooper, of course, had informed me of what would take place, but I wasn't prepared to see it. As I looked down and tried to compose myself before it was my turn to speak, Dr. Rita Snow, who was sitting behind me, whispered, "Are you all right, Sherry?"

"Yes, thank you. I'll be fine." I replied.

Doctors, however, are an interesting breed. Not only did they watch the graphic slides, but they continued to eat their lunch unaffected. (Kind of like *I* would eat popcorn watching a romantic comedy.)

When Dr. Cooper completed his presentation, he gave me a warm introduction. With my knees knocking from fright, I went up to the front. I started by sharing a recent newspaper article about a woman in New Mexico. She feared that the breast implants she received after her bilateral mastectomy were making her ill. Her insurance refused to pay for their removal, and since she didn't have the money to pay a surgeon, she used a razor and removed the silicone gel herself. She did this desperate act one day after visiting a plastic surgeon to learn how it was done.

Waiting until her husband and three children had gone to bed, she used a makeshift scalpel that she had fashioned from a disposable razor. She kept her shaking to a minimum with the use of Valium. She squeezed the silicone gel from the first implant but wasn't able to remove the plastic bag that had held the gel. After going to bed for a while, she got up and attempted to remove the other implant. The next day, a doctor removed the plastic bags in his office.

As I told this story, some nodded their heads as they remembered reading about it themselves; others gasped at the horror of hearing it for the first time. I remarked that this act was extremely foolish at best, but it illustrated very graphically the fear some women are experiencing because of the current implant controversy. It also demonstrates an urgent need for doctors to inform their patients of another option, an option that my personal experience showed to be a far better, healthier one.

I tried to convey to the group the diversity in women's opinions and feelings about the need for reconstruction. I emphasized what a personal choice it was and that all three options—no reconstruction, implant, or autogenous (from one's own body) tissue—needed to be presented to their patients at the time of cancer diagnosis, so that women would be able to have the opportunity, and time, to decide on their best personal option.

I concluded by expressing how grateful I was to Dr. Cooper. His skill not only helped me physically, but emotionally as well. I stressed how fortunate we were to have him in Spokane, so available to us, and urged them one last time to tell their patients.

Whew, to have that over was such a relief! Dr. Cooper and I decided to talk later to determine how we could polish the presentation for the following week at the Women's Health Network.

He called later that afternoon, and as we hashed over the meeting, asked for my input. My only suggestion was that the graphic slides could perhaps be eliminated when we present to women's groups. If I had seen those before my surgery, they may have even scared *me* off, and they might certainly "gross out" another potential candidate.

I asked him to critique my portion of the meeting. He said he thought it was good but asked me not to praise him so much. I apologized for making him uncomfortable, explaining that my heartfelt gratitude is a difficult thing to suppress. He said he understood but asked me to please try.

I adjusted my presentation to fit an audience primarily of women. Although I was still a bit nervous, the next presentation wasn't quite so traumatic for me. Jerry, Donna, and Lynn were sitting there smiling at me and thinking about all I had been through, beginning with my diagnosis and continuing right up to that moment. They thought of that meeting as a graduation of sorts and the launching of a new ministry. It was a confirmation that God's word had once again been proven to be true. He doesn't allow His children to suffer without a purpose.

The meeting went well and at its conclusion Deanna introduced herself and her friend Cindy to me. Deanna had already had a mastectomy and was considering reconstruction. Several of my friends attended her church and had excitedly told Deanna about my reconstruction and put us in touch with each other. We spoke on the telephone and I invited her to come to the meeting so she could find out more about the surgery and meet Dr. Cooper. When we met that evening, she related to me that she had already made her appointment with Dr. Cooper and would be seeing him the following week. I sensed a special warmth and enthusiasm in Deanna that drew me to her.

It turned out that while Dr. Cooper was in the midst of Deanna's reconstruction, he found more cancer. After consulting with Deanna's husband, Dan, Dr. Cooper removed all of the cancer and finished the surgery. A recuperation period followed, and then Deanna began chemotherapy treatments. The chemotherapy thinned her hair, but she was happy she didn't loose it completely. Deanna was once again on the road to recovery, enjoying life with her husband and their children and continuing her church activities and her job as a school bus driver.

Deanna's friend Cindy called me a few months after the Women's Health Network Seminar. Thanking me for my part in the seminar, she confessed that she never would have attended if Deanna hadn't requested her company. Cindy felt that if you were not personally dealing with breast cancer, you wouldn't necessarily pay attention to the reconstructive options available. I agreed that had I not been dealing with it, I most probably wouldn't have given it much thought myself. She was grateful to know about the Free TRAM Flap option, realizing that being informed at a time when you're *not* dealing with it is a real advantage. She asked me to speak at a Wednesday night women's meeting at their church, feeling that this was news worth spreading. I agreed and we set a date.

Cindy and I found ourselves becoming "fast friends" over the telephone—you name it, we talked about it. The scheduled women's meeting was canceled because of a snowstorm. We rescheduled and continued our new friendship over the telephone. I confided to her a lame-brained idea I was getting about writing a book, with the hope that I could reach more women with information about this surgery. She surprised me with an enthusiasm that startled me, almost insisting that I follow through.

I had been fighting this cockeyed book notion for months. Whenever it popped into my head I would say, "Get serious Lord. I can't write a book! After all, I have no experience or training. A person can't just start writing a book, you know! First of all, you have to be really smart, and really smart I ain't! Second, you need to be a grammar expert, a scholar, or some other highfalutin' kinda person. I'm just a homemaker, a domestic goddess. Cleaning toilets is my life (especially since the house majority happens to be male-type people). Besides that, I'm too busy. For instance, after Bible study today I have lunch with the girls (next to cleaning toilets, lunch is my life!). And tomorrow I'm going to buy gum, paint my toenails, and watch Oprah! So, as you can see, I rarely have the time to *read* a book. I may be wrong, but I kinda suspect *writing* one just might possibly be a smidgen more challenging."

I wasn't taking this idea too seriously, so the Lord did something *really* pushy—He sicced my friend Torchy on me! He knew that she listened to Him better than I did and that she would come after me with a vengeance. *She* obeyed him. (She's such a show off!)

Torchy invited me to the Northwest Christian Writers' Conference. "What a crazy idea," I argued. "I'm not a writer!" She was persistent, however, so I agreed to ask Jerry. *Of course, I thought, he will tell me that with Michael in college, someone like me who isn't even a writer shouldn't spend money attending a writers' conference. I will have to be a submissive wife and that will take care of that!* (I'd always wanted to rip that submission stuff out of my Bible, but now it just might come in handy!)

I explained to Jerry, "You know this silly book notion that keeps haunting me? Well, Torchy wants me to go to this writers' conference. But, of course, with Michael in college, we probably shouldn't spend the money, right?"

He replied, "I agree with Torchy, Honey. I think you should go!" What a traitor *he* turned out to be!

I took off for the conference, where I not only received lots of encouragement but found out you don't *have* to be a brilliant scholar with perfect grammar. An author of a book can be just a regular-type person who has something to say with someone interested in what they say.

That's me! I thought. I always have stuff to say! I don't always have people interested in what I say, but that's never stopped me before! I do, however, have something worth saying and information people need to hear.

I decided to go downstairs and try to write. To my surprise the words came swiftly (at least that day) and actually made some sense. I am a sanguine, though, and as charming as a sanguine can be, we are not noted for diligent discipline; nor are we famous for finishing a project. So, if this is an actual book that you are holding in your hands, you are witnessing a major miracle.

Time came for me to speak at Cindy's and Deanna's church. The meeting was upstairs in what some call the "Upper Room." (I felt pretty uppity getting to speak in the upper room!) Cindy had done a lot of promoting and was thrilled at the number of ladies who attended. It went very well. Deanna was there, and after the meeting she proudly spoke of her Free TRAM Flap. She looked wonderful.

The "grapevine" was up and running. I was called weekly by someone who had heard about the surgery and wanted me to talk to a friend or a loved one. I was invited to speak to various women's groups, from church groups to Mammography Society meetings. Marianne Mishima, a news anchor on KXLY, did a story that informed her television audience of their options.

I received a call from Toni Robideaux, an experienced writer and a breast cancer survivor who had been asked by the American Cancer Society to put together an insert for the local newspaper. This insert was to appear on October 1, 1993, to kick off "Breast Cancer Awareness Month." Toni asked if she could do my story, and as we talked, she discovered that I was writing a book. She surprised me by asking me to write my own story. I was honored. It was good experience for me and I learned a lot. Toni was the first professional writer who actually called *me* a writer. I'll always be grateful to her for allowing me that experience. Thanks to many women, and some men as well, who took the news and ran with it. The good news was finally being told. Women were becoming aware of their third option—at least, on a small scale.

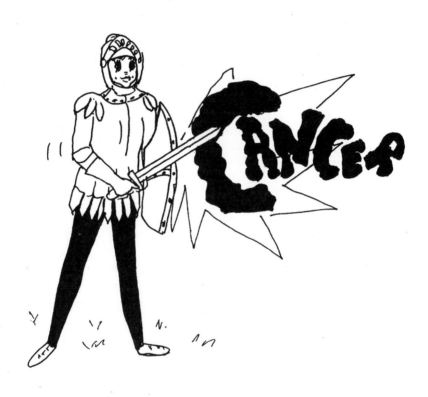

Chapter Seventeen

It's a War Out There!

In the spring, Deanna and Cindy invited me to their women's retreat. I was hesitant because of my family schedule; but, they were persistent, so I agreed to go. Deanna picked up Cindy and me in her van, and as we drove to the church to see if anyone else needed a ride, Cindy and I fussed over Deanna's new pixie haircut. We were soon on the road, headed for Pinelow Nazarene Campground on Deer Lake. The three of us shared a room, and we had a blast. We enjoyed delicious food and a great speaker— even the weather cooperated. Laughter abounded. We took walks and talked into the wee morning hours, when I finally pooped out on them.

The next morning Deanna and I went to take a shower while Cindy caught a few more winks. I hollered over the barrier between our shower stalls, "Deanna, I betcha this is the first time in the history of the world that two TRAM Flappers have showered together!"

She laughed, "You're probably right!"

Deanna mentioned several times during our weekend that her shoulder was bothering her. She'd been to the doctor, and it was decided that her pain was the result of being rear-ended in a car accident. The accident had been in February, however, and she thought it was odd that in May the pain was increasing instead of decreasing.

After our weekend, Deanna's pain worsened. Her doctor prescribed pain medication, and she began seeking other forms of relief by seeing a chiropractor and a massage therapist. When she related to her doctor that nothing was helping and she needed a stronger pain medication, he declined and suggested she see a counselor. Her frustrated husband, Dan, took her to see another doctor and within weeks of our retreat, Deanna was diagnosed with cancer once again.

I relished calling my neighbor Liane "The Boss of the Neighborhood." She was in charge of "Block Watch" and watched over the neighborhood with loving concern. As a young German girl she had married Gary, an American G.I., and had accompanied him to America. They settled in Spokane to raise their family, a daughter and a son. Liane, too, was a victim of breast cancer. She took daily walks and was trying to regain her health.

She came over one afternoon to deliver the "Block Watch Newsletter." During her visit, she revealed that the cancer was back and she was going through chemotherapy again. As she left, she turned to me and said, "It's probably going to get me eventually, but I'm going to put up a fight!"

I was numb. My friend Deanna, and now my neighbor Liane.

I kept posted on Deanna through Cindy and on Liane through my neighbor Carol. I prayed for them, but when I thought of going to see them, I seemed to be paralyzed. Deanna and I were the same age, and Liane was just a bit older. It was too close. I couldn't deal with it.

I finally got up the courage to go to see Liane. Carol and I went together. Liane was struggling just to speak to us; even so, we had a sweet time together. She wanted to be released from the body that had turned against her, but she was waiting. She held on because her brother was on this way from Germany. She wanted to see him one more time, and she did.

My neighbors, Carol and Donna, came to see me at dusk one day in August of 1993. Jerry was working late that night, and I was thrilled to have some company—until I realized they were coming to tell me that Liane had just died.

The neighborhood decided to have a tree planted at her church in her memory. The pine tree is just over her back fence. We all drive past it daily. It's a beautiful reminder to us of a lovely lady.

When I returned home from Liane's funeral, I sat on the couch and cried my eyes out. That evening I was depressed and noticed my heart beating strangely: it would miss a beat and then thump hard. After taking my pulse, Jerry called the doctor. The doctor on call asked if I was under any stress. Jerry explained what I was going through, and the doctor said it probably was stress; but it wouldn't hurt to have an EKG.

The EKG revealed an occasional irregular rhythm, premature ventricular contractions, brought on by fear. I feared, that the enemy, cancer—which in its heartless, evil, cruelty had killed Liane—would ambush me again.

Then in October of 1993, Deanna lost her battle, or should I say graduated from this life into heavenly, everlasting life. Deanna's memorial service was a celebration of her life, with not only tears but much laughter as Pastor Denny read tributes to Deanna written by her friends.

Even when the cancer in your body has been removed, there is a haunting residue left behind. It's a kind of cancer paranoia, but someone who hasn't walked the walk may have a difficult time understanding why the aches and pains that weren't given a second thought before are now the cause of great anxiety.

When you lose the friends with whom you were fighting side by side in the trenches, you not only grieve for them, but you identify with them. Like men in war who have watched the buddy beside them die and wondered why they themselves were spared, you, likewise, wonder. You feel guilt and gratitude at the same time. You fear that the next battle will be yours, that you will also be a casualty in the ugly war cancer has declared—and has too often won. Your heart breaks at the thought of your family struggling along without you. The very idea is unbearable.

I was listening to the radio one morning when I heard Anne Frahm being interviewed. Anne's cancer began as two little lumps in her breast and spread throughout her body. Tumors were found covering her skull, her shoulder, her ribs, her pelvic bone, and up and down her spine.

For a year and a half, Anne underwent every conventional therapy, surgery, chemotherapy, radiation, and hormone therapy. Finally, she underwent an autologous bone marrow transplant. None of these conventional treatments sent her cancer into remission.

"The medical world pronounced me 'hopeless,'" Anne says, "and I was not ready to lie down and play dead."

Early in her cancer battle, she had gone to the library and devoured every book she could find on breast cancer. Anne noticed that some of them, "coldly sang my funeral dirge." She returned them to the shelves and focused on the books that had stories of various individuals who had overcome every form of cancer there was. Some had even made it back to life from their deathbed. She took the encouragement she found in these books, teamed it with her own resolve to be an overcomer, and decided to fight her enemy with every ounce of her being.

When the traditional weapons of war against her cancer proved ineffective, her doctors said they had done all they could and she was sent home—to die.

The medical profession had clearly given up on her; she, however, wasn't ready to give up. She was only thirty-five and had a family to raise, so she decided to "give the nutritional approach another shot." Anne had read about the link between cancer and diet and in fact had seen a nutritionist earlier in her war, but she had been reluctant to make the changes that were suggested. This time she was ready to fight.

Under the guidance of a nutritional counselor, she began a strict regimen of detoxification, diet, and supplements. Five weeks later, tests done by her oncologist revealed no trace of cancer!

She and her husband, David, have written a book on her amazing journey. Their book is entitled *A Cancer Battle Plan*. I believe it is one of the most, if not *the* most, important books written in our "cancer epidemic" time. Their wonderful book is a condensed version of all they have learned about beating cancer in the face of little medical hope. Their strategy for fighting this deadly nemesis is:

1. Know your enemy
2. Cut off enemy supply lines
3. Rebuild your natural defense system
4. Bring in reinforcements
5. Maintain morale
6. Carefully select your professional help

They have researched data, condensed it, and explained it in Anne's easy-to-read, personal story. It illustrates that not only our family history, but our toxic environment and diet play a serious role. They have explained what to do, how to do it, and why.

141

Anne and David have also started a nonprofit organization called *HealthQuarters*, through which they send out a newsletter filled with information, education, and encouragement.

To receive *HealthQuarters Newsletter* or more information write:

HealthQuarters
6873 Prince Drive
Colorado Springs, Co. 80918

I had the honor and pleasure of meeting Anne when she was in Spokane to share her story of faith, hope, and nutrition. We talked about our cancer battle and my reconstruction. I asked, and she graciously granted me, permission to share her story in this book.

As I write this, Anne and David are in the process of launching their dream, *HealthQuarters Lodge*, which will be a health retreat in the mountains of Colorado. At their "health get-away," people will not only be taught the principles of nutrition but will actually work on their health with the help of professionals. Their guests will receive:

- A full nutritional analysis and monitoring by a certified nutritionist
- A program of foods and supplements tailored to their specific nutritional analysis
- Three meals a day based upon their unique nutritional needs
- Two massages a week by a professional massage therapist
- Two colonic treatments a week (water irrigation of the bowel) by a professional colonic therapist
- Instructional classes and demonstrations
- Encouragement and prayers
- Networking assistance to find like-minded people and professionals "back home"

- Transportation to and from the airport

They do caution that they are an educational and self-help center, not a hospital. Their retreat center will not be for everyone. If you are too sick to help yourself, or don't have a friend to come along to help, their lodge is not for you. They also will not practice medicine or prescribe drugs.

Their goals are to teach people who are fighting cancer, "cancer cousins," how to detoxify their bodies, give their immune systems the tools they need to fight disease, and render emotional and spiritual encouragement.

I strongly urge anyone who wants to declare war on cancer to invest in Anne and David Frahm's book, *A Cancer Battle Plan.*

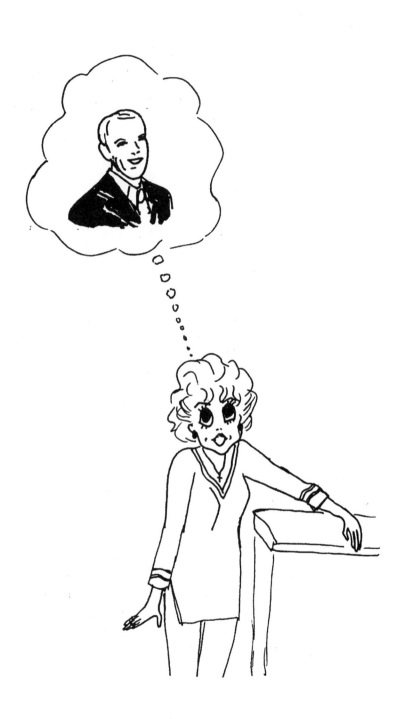

Chapter Eighteen

Heroes

Ann Jillian has been kind of a hero to me. I have always thought her beautiful and talented, and I admire her spirit. When her breast cancer was made public, I grieved with her. How would such a beautiful, sexy woman deal emotionally with the loss of her breasts? She chose to have no reconstruction long before the silicone implant controversy. I was amazed by her self-confidence and boldness. When the movie about her cancer experience was on television, I went through all of the emotions with her. I never suspected that I would someday experience the same emotions myself. The courage she exhibited by portraying herself—submitting herself to that intense pain all over again—amazed me.

I saw her on a talk show, and I remember her sharing the strength she received from her husband, Andy, as they went through that valley in their lives together. She asked him to come out on the set and join her. He sat on a stool next to hers, and she sang him a love song that came straight from her heart. It permanently pierced mine. It was called, "Wind Beneath My Wings." It was a privilege to watch Ann's touching musical tribute to her husband, and it deeply moved me. As I listened to her sing, I realized that she was putting into words what Jerry has meant to me.

I am the extrovert, the one who gets the attention. Jerry is the strong, silent type. One of the phrases in the song says, "You were content to let me shine; that's your way. You always walked a step behind." That's Jerry. He stands back and lovingly watches as I *work the crowd*, the crowd being one or one hundred in number.

A sanguine is a peculiar creature who can be down in the dumps one minute, but walk into a roomful of people and "It's show time!" Something just magically happens—most of the time.

I went through a time in my life when I was uncomfortable with that part of my personality. I longed to be a demure sophisticate, an intellectual able to converse with a nuclear scientist, and with little or no effort, to dazzle him or her with my brilliance. I would try at times to reach that goal, but the effort usually would or could only last about ten minutes. It was hopeless! I have finally come to realize that it's unlikely that I will ever become a sophisticated intellectual. *Cerebral* will never be an adjective used to describe me. Finally, I'm becoming comfortable being Sherry Lynn, the hopeless nut who sees things in life through an unconventional kaleidoscope. You can't buy this bizarre kaleidoscope. You are born with it. Either it's there, or it ain't. If you don't have one, it's quite possible you may wonder if the ones who *do* are missing something upstairs. The truth is, nothing is missing; some of us just have something extra—a kaleidoscope! (I wonder if one has ever shown up on a brain scan?)

Sanguines are *very* serious about their fun! A "normal" person would consider that statement to be an oxymoron—a sanguine finds it truth. Patsy Clairmont's second book is called, *Normal Is Just a Setting on Your Dryer.* I *love* that title! Normal?

Who wants to be normal? Let's try for extraordinary! At the very least, let's shoot for above-normal. I no longer wish to be normal. Especially since synonyms for normal include: average, common, ordinary, and typical. Bo-o-oring! I have finally reached a point in my life where I am content about being born with something "normal" people don't have. I am dedicated to fun and I love to get a laugh, especially from someone who looks like they've been suckin' on a dill pickle!

One reason I have finally come to terms with myself is partly because it just seems to happen to a woman about the time she's ambushed by mid-life. In my case, however, it's mostly because of Jerry. He is *more* than comfortable with who I am. As a matter of fact, I can practically do no wrong. (Well, there *was* that time when he was at the ranch with his dad and brother, Ken. His bladder was about to burst, and he discovered that I had sewn up the fly in his boxer shorts; but he got over it! He and his dad plotted revenge and decided it would be great to tie my pantyhose in multiple knots! It's very difficult to put pantyhose on around all those knots, and my legs looked quite lumpy!)

Jerry is definitely the "Wind Beneath my Wings," the one who enables me to soar as Sherry Lynn. I am eternally grateful for the freedom and encouragement he gives to me. As the song says, "It might have appeared to go unnoticed; but, I have it all here in my heart. I want you to know, I know the truth, of course, I know. My life would be empty without you."

In September of 1992, I spoke at three Christian Women's Club meetings in Montana. The last one was in Eureka, a small town by the Canadian border. They put on a wonderful luncheon and fashion show. Before I spoke, the vocalist sang "Wind Beneath My Wings." I was tired from the trip, missing Jerry, and anxious to get home to him. Before I knew it, I was tearing up. I pictured in my mind Ann Jillian singing that song to her husband, Andy. I was reminded of Ann's and my mutual struggle with breast cancer. I thought of my husband and his loyalty, love, and the strength he gave me as he helped me to face cancer. When you are sitting at the head table, unable either to hide the silent, trickling tears or to crawl under the table without people noticing, you have a dilemma. I managed to pull myself together before my turn at the mike. When I came to the part in my story about the cancer, I explained about Ann Jillian and about how her song to her husband became my song to mine. "Someday," I told them, "I might be able to listen to it without a tug at my heart, but I'm not there yet." I think they understood.

I don't have many heroes on this earth. Roy Rogers, the ultimate "good guy" and my hero since childhood, whom, to my *extreme*, never-ending delight, I had the privilege of meeting face to face; Ann Jillian, a beautiful woman who handled her breast cancer with style, grace, and humor; and Jerry, my real hero, my husband. To Jerry I would like to say, "Did I ever tell you you're my hero? You're everything I'd like to be. I can fly higher than an eagle, for you are the wind beneath my wings!"

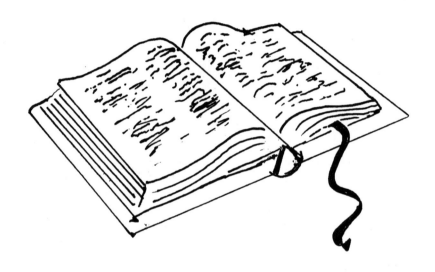

Chapter Nineteen
The Really Good News!

I was compelled to write this book to spread the "good news" about a little known breast reconstructive option which is available. I also hoped to make the reader chuckle a little, and perhaps, in some small way, to take a bit of the sting out of the ugly experience of cancer. I wanted to show that humor can help even the biggest yellowbellied pantywaist of all time, *me*, cope with an immense and overwhelming trial.

The concept of writing this book also brought with it an enormous dilemma. When it was being formed in my mind, I struggled, wondering whether or not I would reach more women if I addressed my cancer encounter and reconstruction only, excluding the spiritual part of my struggle. I didn't want this to be a book exclusively for Christian women because breast cancer, reconstruction, and the like, are issues that touch women with diverse opinions and beliefs. I would like every woman to know of this wonderful option.

Through my struggle I finally realized that to describe this episode in my life without mentioning the Lord's presence would be like writing about my marriage and neglecting to mention Jerry's presence. I couldn't do it.

Some of you are rolling your eyes now saying, "Here it comes, the religious pitch." To those of you who feel that way, I give permission to close the book at this point if you like. I won't be offended if you just take the "good news" about the reconstruction, along with my hopefully interesting and sometimes humorous account, and call chapter eighteen the conclusion of my book. However, I would be remiss if I neglected to explain to whom I was writing in my journal, who walked through the valley of cancer with me, who it is that I call Lord. If I didn't write this chapter, perhaps you would miss the even more wonderful "good news."

It may be a relief for you to know that I am not going to tell you about "religion." Religion is only man's feeble attempt to reach God. This attempt is, and has always been, unnecessary. Man didn't have to drum up "religion" in order to fill the empty hole in the soul. God Himself has done the work, and I for one, am thankful! Religions are *so* confusing, being as many in number as M & M's in a big bag of candy. A person could strip a gear in his or her brain trying to find the right one. The fact that there *are* so many only proves that there is a void in the very center of our being, and we have a longing to fill it with something.

What I have is not a religion. What I have is a relationship with a constant companion, a loving comforter, a Savior. He is as real to me as the computer I am using to write this book. How can that be? You can see and touch a computer; once more, you have to pay big bucks for a computer. That *really* makes *it* real.

According to Hebrews 11:1, "Now faith is being sure of what we hope for and certain of what we do not see." *That* is a toughie. How can someone believe something they can't see? It seems like a peculiar concept, yet we do it every day. We pick up the telephone, believing there will be a person on the line, a person we cannot see. We have faith that the gravity we cannot see will always be there and that when we get out of bed in the morning we won't float around the room like an astronaut.

We, as people, are so complex; we seem to be born self-centered. Even a child who has been taught impeccable manners will snatch a toy from another child's hands and squeal, *"Mine!"* Children don't have to be taught to bite someone, lie, or take something that doesn't belong to them. On the contrary, they have to be taught that these natural inclinations are wrong.

Who we are as adults is determined, in part, by what we have experienced since birth. Our experiences affect how we view life, how we view people, how we view God. Our most painful experiences sometimes spawn less than favorable reactions. When we have suffered a wrong, whether it is real or how we perceived the incident (a misunderstanding), we want to strike out in anger, or pain—we want revenge. Maybe not revenge in the form of taking action against someone, though some do, but also anger turned inward. This comes out in various destructive ways: depression, substance abuse, slander, unforgiveness, trying to control others because you fear what will happen if you don't, etc. The joy in life slips away, eventually bitterness sets in, and your heart becomes hard and cynical. Life is not always a bowl of cherries, and sometimes our reactions to the pits in life become sin. Not only sin against others, but also against ourselves, and most of all, against God.

The God I have faith in is a holy God who hates sin, so our sinful nature is unacceptable to Him. As parents we teach our children that there are consequences for their wayward actions. Likewise, sin carries consequences. Sometimes the consequences we pay are temporal, but they are also eternal. Since God is holy and can't tolerate sin, the price we pay for our sin is death, which at the very least is both a spiritual and eternal separation from Him.

The first part of Romans 6:23 states, "For the wages of sin is death. . . ." Whether we like it or not, there are always consequences for actions, and if we had to pay the consequences for our sins, we would be doomed!

You may be concluding that God must be a heartless ogre to set us up for the impossible task of accomplishing a sinless life, and then punishing us forever for something that is naturally in us. Yes, He would be a bit of an ogre had He left it at that and not provided a solution, one that He will extend to anyone who asks. Jesus was the solution; when He died on the cross, He paid the penalty for my sin and your sin. Because of His holiness, God cannot look upon sin. Jesus was sinless, and because of who He was and is (the God-Man), His payment was satisfying to God, allowing God to remain just and holy and still accept sinful man into His family. Jesus suffered our punishment, and because of Him, our debt is canceled; it's marked "Paid in full."

When I was a little girl, my brother, Brett, used to bite himself and tell our parents that I bit him. I really resented being unjustly punished, but think of it: Jesus accepted our punishment, being fully innocent, and He did it without resentment.

I believed as a child that Pontius Pilate was a horrible and mean man who murdered Jesus, the Son of God. In fact, history records that Pilate made efforts to release Jesus, perceiving that he was an innocent man. Pilate, a politician, only succumbed to the pressure of an angry mob. Jesus wasn't a victim, however, because He knew what He was facing and did it willingly for our sake. Being God's Son, He could have stopped it. He could have zapped them all on the spot. His love for us made Him choose to go through with it.

The second part of Romans 6:23 states, ". . . but the gift of God is eternal life in Christ Jesus our Lord." God doesn't want our sin to separate us from Him. He loves us and He created us to love Him. Everyone knows that you can't force someone to love you, and who would want to? Love has to be given freely. God knew this and didn't want to force us to love Him, so He gave us a will of our own. I am blessed that Jerry loves me of his own free will and wants to be with me; if I had to force him, his body might be at home with me, but his heart would not, and I would receive no joy from that. God loves us and wants us to return His love freely.

I heard an analogy once about a little boy whose daddy bought him an ant farm. He spent day and night watching the ants. He loved to watch them diligently work, going about their daily ant business. He loved these ants so much that one day he went to his father.

He said, "Daddy, do you think they know that I love them? Oh Daddy, I wish I could somehow tell them and show them how much they mean to me."

His daddy thought for a minute and said, "Son, the only way that would be possible would be if you could, by some miracle, become like them. If you could become an ant, you could go and live among them and show and tell them how much you love them."

In a sense, that is exactly what God did. He became a man so that He could live among us to tell us and show us by His sacrifice the depth of His love for us.

It's a historical fact that Jesus lived and walked on this earth; none may deny that. I know that some can accept Him as a good man, a wonderful teacher, an example for us to pattern our lives after, but not His claim to be God.

To draw from the book, *Mere Christianity*, written by one-time agnostic C. S. Lewis (subject of the wonderful movie *Shadowlands*):

> "A man who was merely a man and said the sort of things Jesus said would not be a great moral teacher. He would either be a lunatic, on the level with a man who says he is a poached egg, . . . or else he would be the devil of hell. You must make your choice. Either this man was, and is, the Son of God or else a madman or something worse. You can shut Him up for a fool . . . or demon; or you can fall at His feet and call Him Lord and God. But let us not come up with any patronizing nonsense about His being a great human teacher. He has not left that alternative open to us. He did not intend to."

It seems there are only three choices here:

1) Jesus was a lunatic who believed His own claims to be God.

2) Jesus knew He wasn't what He claimed and was a deliberately deceitful liar, the ultimate of con men.
3) He was and is who He professed to be while on earth.

It *is* a fact that Jesus Christ lived on this earth, and we all must make an individual choice—lunatic, liar, or Lord.

I do realize that my conviction comes from my belief that the Bible is the word of God. I also realize that someone who does not see the Bible as an authority will think literal belief in it is strange, utter nonsense. That is no surprise to God. 1 Corinthians 1:18 states, "For the message of the cross is foolishness to those who are perishing, but to us who are being saved it is the power of God" (NIV).

Nonbelievers will perhaps see the Bible as a nice book of stories, with a lot of stuff that doesn't make too much sense. They don't take it seriously and have difficulty fathoming why other people do. That is understandable because insight into the Bible takes more than just reading skills. Unfortunately, what it takes cannot be acquired until one has surrendered to the truth of it.

Once you commit your life to Jesus Christ, you receive discernment from the Spirit of God. 1 Corinthians 2:14 states, "The man without the Spirit does not accept the things that come from the Spirit of God, for they are foolishness to him, and he cannot understand them, because they are spiritually discerned" (NIV). Even with this discernment, a Christian (least of all Me) doesn't understand everything in the Bible. But lack of understanding doesn't make it untrue.

I don't, for the life of me, understand a fax machine. It blows my mind that I can put in a sheet of paper, dial a telephone number, my sheet of paper goes through the fax and comes out the other side, and it can be sent across the world—without ever leaving my possession, *Amazing!* My lack of understanding of *how* it works *or* my lack of desire to dig in and learn the mechanics of *why* it works doesn't change the fact that *it works*.

The reality of Christ and the Bible does not change because an individual does or does not believe. If a person does not believe in the concept of gravity and jumps off an eighteen-story building, what he does or does not believe doesn't make any difference. The reality is that he will be introduced to the ground abruptly, and by that time it's too late to have a change of heart and mind. Likewise, if he doesn't believe in the truth of the Bible and what it says regarding eternal destination, upon the death of his body, it will be too late to have a change of heart and mind.

In my observations, there are two kinds of people in particular who have the most difficult time accepting the validity of the Bible. People, who through their talent and abilities have become self-made sometimes see no need to surrender to God, thinking they have done very well putting their faith in themselves. The others are those who find their intellect getting in the way. They want tangible proof. If you who are reading my book fit either of these descriptions, I would like to suggest three things.

1) Read *Mere Christianity* by C. S. Lewis. He was a professor at Cambridge University and an intellectual, a former agnostic who studied the Bible to prove it wrong.
2) Read Josh McDowell's *Evidence That Demands a Verdict,* a compilation of his notes prepared for his lecture series; *Christianity: Hoax or History?* or, his easier to read book, *More Than a Carpenter.*
3) Pray and ask God to reveal Himself to you. Something simple like this: "Lord, if you are real, take the scales off of my eyes so that I might see you. Make yourself real to me. Amen."

If you are sincere, stand back and watch Him work. The reason I suggest this is found in Jeremiah 29: 12–13, "Then you will call upon me and come and pray to me, and I will listen to you. You will seek me and find me when you seek me with all your heart." He is a gentleman who won't force Himself on anyone, but He truly wants to be found by you.

There are some who are under the false assumption that being a moral person, attending church regularly, living by the "golden rule," and not robbing espresso stands, is the correct formula that will favorably determine their eternal destination. Going to church doesn't make someone a Christian any more than going to McDonald's converts them into a hamburger. God really doesn't care what building we go to. There are no denominations in heaven. The denominations, in which some of us take pride, don't impress Him one bit. He only cares about the condition of our hearts and what we do about the sacrifice of His beloved Son, which He made on our behalf. Unfortunately, churches are filled with people who don't know the Lord but who think they are fine because they attend church regularly and sit in their favorite pew listening to a sermon.

Some believe if you can do wonderful things for humanity, surely, this would find favor in God's eyes. Granted, humanity needs a lot of help, and we certainly should do our part; but, it's not a ticket to heaven. It's carefully explained in Ephesians 2:8–9: "For it is by grace you have been saved, through faith—and this not from yourselves, it is the gift of God—not by works, so that no one can boast." This means that faith in Christ is the only way to be made right with God. No human effort can contribute to one's salvation, no matter how noble and good. Once we have that relationship with Him, however, He will motivate us to serve Him, and others will benefit from our service to Him.

It's amazing that something so significant, can be so uncomplicated. It's a gift, and in order for a gift to become yours, you merely reach out and take possession.

This gift of salvation is simply a transaction that takes place in your heart, and no one knows your heart but you and God. And He knows it better than you do.

When you accept the deity of Christ, admit that you in your humanness are a sinner, ask forgiveness for your sins, turn away from your sins, and accept the gift of forgiveness, you have assurance of eternal life.

Involvement in a *Christ-centered, Bible teaching* church is essential. First, it offers assistance in studying the Bible, which is God's love letter to His people and the key to our spiritual growth. It's through Bible study that we, as my friend Donna says, "Change, grow, and become who God created us to be." Second, Jesus instructed us to follow His example in baptism. We need to be obedient to His command. Third, heartfelt relationships with like-minded people are a true gift from the Lord. In my struggle with cancer, my friends couldn't change my circumstances, but the Lord used them to lift my spirits with their love—and that, dear ones, has more value than the purest gold.

A funny thing about God is that He doesn't always pick those whom the world would consider to be important or outstanding people. He often picks people who are not thought of as any big deal, that through working in their lives, He is clearly seen. That is the case with me. I, in myself, am no big deal. I am only a wife and mother who fervently loves her three men. I know that some who don't know me well see me primarily as someone who likes to have fun, which, in part, is who I am. This book just might surprise them a bit, and that's okay; in fact, it's what I want, because then they, too, will see the power of God.

To paraphrase and personalize Ephesians 3:8, "Although I am less than the least of all God's people, this grace was given me: to write this book and share His love."